Table Of Contents

Chapter 1: Understanding the Importance of Lifestyle Change

The Benefits of Making a Lifestyle Change

Making a lifestyle change can be daunting, especially for those who feel stuck in a rut or lack motivation. However, the benefits of making a lifestyle change far outweigh the challenges that may come with it. By taking the first step towards improving your health and well-being, you can experience a whole range of positive outcomes that will not only help you lose weight, but also keep it off for good.

One of the key benefits of making a lifestyle change is the improvement in overall health and fitness. By incorporating regular exercise and healthy eating habits into your daily routine, you can reduce your risk of developing chronic diseases such as diabetes, heart disease, and obesity. In addition, you will also experience increased energy levels, improved mood, and better sleep quality, all of which contribute to a better quality of life.

Another benefit of making a lifestyle change is the positive impact it can have on your mental health. Exercise has been proven to reduce symptoms of depression and anxiety, as well as improve cognitive function and overall brain health. By making time for physical activity and self-care, you can boost your confidence and self-esteem, leading to a more positive outlook on life.

Furthermore, making a lifestyle change can also improve your relationships with others. When you prioritize your health and well-being, you are better equipped to handle the stresses and challenges that come with daily life. This can lead to healthier and more fulfilling relationships with your family, friends, and colleagues, as you are able to show up as your best self both physically and emotionally.

Overall, the benefits of making a lifestyle change are endless. Whether you are looking to lose weight, improve your fitness level, or simply feel better overall, taking small steps towards a healthier lifestyle can have a big impact on your life. By incorporating exercise, healthy eating habits, and self-care into your daily routine, you can experience a transformation that will not only help you reach your goals, but also maintain them for the long term. So why wait? Start making positive changes today and reap the rewards of a healthier, happier you.

Common Barriers to Lifestyle Change

Making a lifestyle change, especially when it comes to losing weight and keeping it off, can be a challenging journey for many individuals. There are several common barriers that can hinder progress and make it difficult to achieve long-term success. In this subchapter, we will explore some of the most common obstacles that people face when trying to make positive lifestyle changes.

One of the most common barriers to lifestyle change is lack of motivation. Many individuals may start off with good intentions, but quickly lose steam when faced with the challenges of making significant changes to their daily routines. This lack of motivation can stem from a variety of factors, such as feeling overwhelmed by the prospect of making changes, or not seeing immediate results from their efforts.

Another common barrier to lifestyle change is being stuck in a rut. This can happen when individuals get into a routine that is comfortable and familiar, even if it is not conducive to their goals. Breaking out of this rut can be difficult, as it often requires stepping outside of one's comfort zone and trying new things.

For many Moms, Dads, and individuals trying to lose weight and keep it off, a lack of support can also be a significant barrier to making positive lifestyle changes. Without a strong support system in place, it can be easy to become discouraged and give up on one's goals. Finding supportive friends, family members, or even online communities can help individuals stay motivated and accountable on their journey.

In addition to lack of motivation, being stuck in a rut, and lack of support, other common barriers to lifestyle change include unrealistic expectations, fear of failure, and negative self-talk. It is important for individuals to recognize these barriers and work towards overcoming them in order to achieve their goals.

By understanding and addressing these common barriers to lifestyle change, individuals can set themselves up for success and create lasting, positive changes in their lives. With determination, perseverance, and a willingness to overcome obstacles, anyone can achieve their weight loss and lifestyle goals.

Setting Realistic Goals for Weight Loss

Setting realistic goals for weight loss is a crucial step in achieving long-term success in your journey towards a healthier lifestyle. For many individuals, especially busy moms, dads, and people struggling to lose weight and keep it off, it can be challenging to stay motivated and focused on their goals. However, by following a few key strategies, you can set achievable goals that will keep you on track and help you reach your desired weight.

One of the first steps in setting realistic goals for weight loss is to establish a clear understanding of your current health and fitness level. This means taking the time to assess your current weight, body measurements, and overall health status. By having a baseline measurement of where you are starting from, you can set specific and attainable goals that are tailored to your individual needs and capabilities.

It is also important to set goals that are realistic and achievable within a reasonable timeframe. For example, instead of setting a goal to lose 20 pounds in a month, which may be unrealistic and unhealthy, consider setting a goal to lose one to two pounds per week. This more gradual approach is not only safer for your body, but also more sustainable in the long run.

In addition to setting realistic weight loss goals, it is important to focus on other aspects of your lifestyle that contribute to your overall health and well-being. This includes incorporating regular physical activity, such as high-intensity interval training (HIIT) workouts, bodyweight exercises, strength training, cardio workouts, yoga, Pilates, or outdoor activities, into your routine. By combining a variety of exercises that you enjoy, you can keep your workouts interesting and challenging, while also promoting weight loss and muscle toning.

While it's important to set a goal for the number of pounds you would like to lose, it's also essential to establish goals for daily and weekly exercise. The amount of time you should dedicate to working out to lose weight can vary depending on factors such as individual goals, current fitness level, and overall health. However, here are some general guidelines: Aim for at least 150 minutes of moderate-intensity aerobic exercise per week: This can include activities such as brisk walking, cycling, swimming, or dancing.

Spread this amount of exercise over several days of the week, aiming for at least 30 minutes of activity on most days. Include strength training exercises at least two days per week: Strength training helps build muscle mass, which can increase metabolism and promote fat loss. Focus on exercises that target major muscle groups, such as squats, lunges, push-ups, and rows.

Listen to your body and gradually increase intensity: If you're new to exercise or have been inactive for a while, start slowly and gradually increase the duration and intensity of your workouts as your fitness level improves. Pay attention to how your body responds to exercise and make adjustments as needed. Remember to include rest days: Rest and recovery are important components of any workout routine, allowing your muscles time to repair and rebuild.

Aim to include at least one or two rest days per week to prevent overtraining and reduce the risk of injury. Ultimately, the key to successful weight loss is finding a balance between diet and exercise that works for you and is sustainable in the long term. It's also important to consult with a healthcare professional before starting any new exercise program, especially if you have any underlying health conditions or concerns.

Another thing to mention when trying to get the required amount of work out time in, is the aid of a workout tool such as a Fitbits or an Apple watch for example. Fitbits, Apple Watches, and similar fitness trackers can be effective tools for weight loss when used in conjunction with a balanced diet and regular exercise routine. Here are some ways these devices can help.

Activity Tracking: Fitbits and Apple Watches can monitor your daily activity levels, including steps taken, distance traveled, and calories burned. By providing real-time feedback on your activity, these devices can motivate you to move more throughout the day and reach your daily activity goals. Heart

Rate Monitoring: Many fitness trackers offer heart rate monitoring capabilities, which can provide valuable information about the intensity of your workouts and help you gauge your overall cardiovascular fitness. Monitoring your heart rate during exercise can also help you optimize your workouts for maximum calorie burn and fitness gains. Goal Setting and Progress Tracking:

Fitness trackers allow you to set personalized fitness goals and track your progress over time. Whether you're aiming to lose weight, improve your endurance, or increase your daily activity levels, these devices can help you stay focused and motivated by visually tracking your progress and celebrating your achievements.

Reminder and Motivation: Some fitness trackers offer features such as reminders to move, workout reminders, and motivational messages to help keep you on track with your fitness goals. These gentle nudges can encourage you to stay active throughout the day and make healthier choices.

Community and Accountability: Many fitness trackers have built-in social features that allow you to connect with friends, join challenges, and share your progress with others. This sense of community and accountability can provide additional motivation and support as you work towards your weight loss goals. While fitness trackers can be valuable tools for weight loss, it's important to remember that they are just one part of the equation. To achieve sustainable weight loss, it's essential to combine regular exercise with a healthy diet, adequate sleep, stress management, and other lifestyle factors. Additionally, it's important to use fitness trackers as a guide rather than relying solely on them for weight loss.

Furthermore, nutrition plays a key role in achieving weight loss goals. By developing a meal plan that is balanced and nutritious, you can fuel your body with the necessary nutrients to support your workouts and promote fat burning. Consider consulting with a nutritionist or dietitian to create a meal plan that aligns with your weight loss goals and dietary preferences.

Ultimately, setting realistic goals for weight loss requires dedication, patience, and a willingness to make sustainable lifestyle changes. By taking a holistic approach to your health and fitness journey, you can set yourself up for long-term success and achieve your desired weight in a healthy and sustainable way. Remember, progress takes time, so be kind to yourself and celebrate even the smallest victories along the way.

Chapter 2: Workout and Weight Loss Guide

Introduction to Different Types of Workouts

If you are someone who is feeling low motivation and stuck in a rut when it comes to working out, you are not alone. Many Moms, Dads, or anyone trying to lose weight and keep it off struggle with finding the right type of workout that fits their lifestyle and goals. In this subchapter, we will explore various types of workouts that can help you kickstart your fitness journey and make lasting changes to your lifestyle.

One popular type of workout that is gaining traction in the fitness world is High-intensity interval training (HIIT) workouts. HIIT involves short bursts of intense exercise followed by brief periods of rest or lower intensity exercise. This type of workout is known for its efficiency in burning calories and improving cardiovascular health, making it a great option for those looking to maximize their workout time.

Bodyweight exercises are another effective way to lose weight and build muscle without the need for any equipment. These exercises, such as push-ups, squats, and planks, can be done anywhere and are great for beginners looking to strengthen their muscles and improve their overall fitness level. By incorporating bodyweight exercises into your routine, you can see significant improvements in your strength and endurance.

For those who are new to strength training, it can be intimidating to navigate the world of weightlifting and resistance training. However, strength training is essential for building muscle, increasing metabolism, and improving overall body composition. By starting with basic exercises and gradually increasing the weight and intensity, beginners can safely and effectively incorporate strength training into their workout routine.

Cardio workouts are often associated with fat burning and weight loss, making them a popular choice for individuals looking to shed excess pounds. Activities such as running, cycling, and swimming can help improve cardiovascular health, boost metabolism, and burn calories. By incorporating cardio workouts into your routine, you can see improvements in your overall fitness level and reach your weight loss goals.

In addition to traditional gym workouts, outdoor workouts can provide a refreshing change of scenery and a boost in motivation. Activities such as hiking, biking, and outdoor boot camps can help you connect with nature, reduce stress, and burn calories in a fun and enjoyable way. By exploring different types of outdoor workouts, you can find a new way to stay active and make lasting changes to your lifestyle.

Finding the Right Workout Routine for You

First and foremost make sure to consult your personal physician to ensure you are healthy enough for a physical workout routine that you select.
Finding the right workout routine for you can be a daunting task, especially if you are feeling low motivated or stuck in a rut. As busy Moms, Dads, or individuals trying to lose weight and keep it off, it can be challenging to know where to start. However, with the right guidance and determination, you can find a workout routine that is not only effective but also enjoyable.

One option to consider is high-intensity interval training (HIIT) workouts. HIIT workouts are known for their ability to burn a significant amount of calories in a short amount of time. This type of workout is perfect for those who are short on time but still want to see results. HIIT workouts can be done at home or in a gym setting, making them a convenient option for busy individuals.

If you prefer bodyweight exercises for weight loss, there are plenty of options to choose from. Bodyweight exercises, such as squats, lunges, and push-ups, can be effective for building muscle and burning fat. These exercises can be done anywhere, without the need for any equipment, making them a great option for those who prefer to workout at home.

Strength training for beginners is another option to consider when looking for the right workout routine. Strength training can help build muscle, increase metabolism, and improve overall strength and endurance. Beginners can start with bodyweight exercises or light weights and gradually increase the intensity as they become more comfortable with the movements.

Cardio workouts for fat burning are essential for those looking to shed excess weight. Whether you prefer running, cycling, or dancing, incorporating cardio into your routine can help boost your metabolism and burn calories. Cardio workouts can be done indoors or outdoors, depending on your preference and availability of space.

In addition to finding the right workout routine, it is essential to focus on nutrition and meal planning for weight loss. Eating a balanced diet that is rich in fruits, vegetables, lean proteins, and whole grains can help support your fitness goals. Working with a nutritionist or dietitian can help you create a meal plan that is tailored to your specific needs and goals.

Overall, finding the right workout routine for you is a personal journey that requires patience, dedication, and perseverance. By exploring different options, such as HIIT workouts, bodyweight exercises, strength training, cardio workouts, and nutrition planning, you can create a routine that works best for your lifestyle and fitness goals. Remember to listen to your body, stay consistent, and seek support from professionals or online communities to help you stay motivated and on track towards achieving your weight loss and lifestyle change goals.

Incorporating Exercise into Your Daily Routine

Incorporating exercise into your daily routine can be a game-changer when it comes to losing weight and keeping it off. For many of us, finding the motivation to workout can be a challenge, especially when we are stuck in a rut or feeling low on energy. However, by making small, manageable changes to your daily routine, you can easily incorporate exercise into your life and start seeing results.

One of the best ways to incorporate exercise into your daily routine is to schedule it like any other appointment or commitment. Set aside a specific time each day for your workout, whether it's early in the morning before the kids wake up, during your lunch break, or in the evening after dinner. By making exercise a priority and scheduling it into your day, you are more likely to stick to it and make it a habit.

Another way to incorporate exercise into your daily routine is to find activities that you enjoy and look forward to. Whether it's going for a walk outside, taking a yoga class, or hitting the gym for a high-intensity interval training (HIIT) workout, finding activities that you enjoy will make it easier to stay motivated and consistent. Remember, exercise doesn't have to be a chore – it can be fun and rewarding!

If you're feeling overwhelmed by the idea of incorporating exercise into your daily routine, start small. Begin with just 10 or 15 minutes of exercise each day, whether it's a quick bodyweight workout, a short walk around the neighborhood, or a few minutes of stretching. As you build up your strength and endurance, you can gradually increase the duration and intensity of your workouts.

Finally, remember that consistency is key when it comes to incorporating exercise into your daily routine. Even on days when you're feeling tired or unmotivated, try to do something active, even if it's just a short walk or some gentle stretching. By staying consistent with your workouts, you will not only see physical results, but you will also feel more energized, confident, and motivated to continue on your weight loss and lifestyle change journey.

Chapter 3: High-Intensity Interval Training (HIIT) Workouts

What is HIIT and How Does it Work?

High-intensity interval training (HIIT) has become a popular workout choice for those looking to lose weight and improve their fitness levels. But what exactly is HIIT, and how does it work? In simple terms, HIIT involves alternating between short bursts of intense exercise and periods of rest or lower-intensity exercise. This method is designed to keep your heart rate up and maximize calorie burn in a short amount of time.

One of the key benefits of HIIT is its ability to boost your metabolism, both during and after your workout. This means that you continue to burn calories even after you've finished exercising, making it an efficient way to lose weight. Additionally, HIIT workouts can help improve your cardiovascular fitness, increase your endurance, and build strength.

For those who may be feeling low motivated or stuck in a rut when it comes to their fitness routine, HIIT can be a game-changer. This type of training is known for its time efficiency, making it ideal for busy parents or individuals with packed schedules. With HIIT, you can get a challenging and effective workout in as little as 20-30 minutes, making it easier to stick to a consistent exercise routine.

Incorporating bodyweight exercises into your HIIT routine can further enhance your weight loss efforts. These exercises, such as squats, lunges, push-ups, and planks, can help build muscle and increase your overall calorie burn. Strength training for beginners is also beneficial for boosting metabolism and toning your body.

Cardio workouts are another essential component of HIIT, as they help maximize fat burning and improve cardiovascular health. Whether you prefer running, cycling, or jumping rope, incorporating cardio intervals into your HIIT routine can help you achieve your weight loss goals. By combining high-intensity intervals with periods of lower intensity or rest, you can push your body to its limits and see results

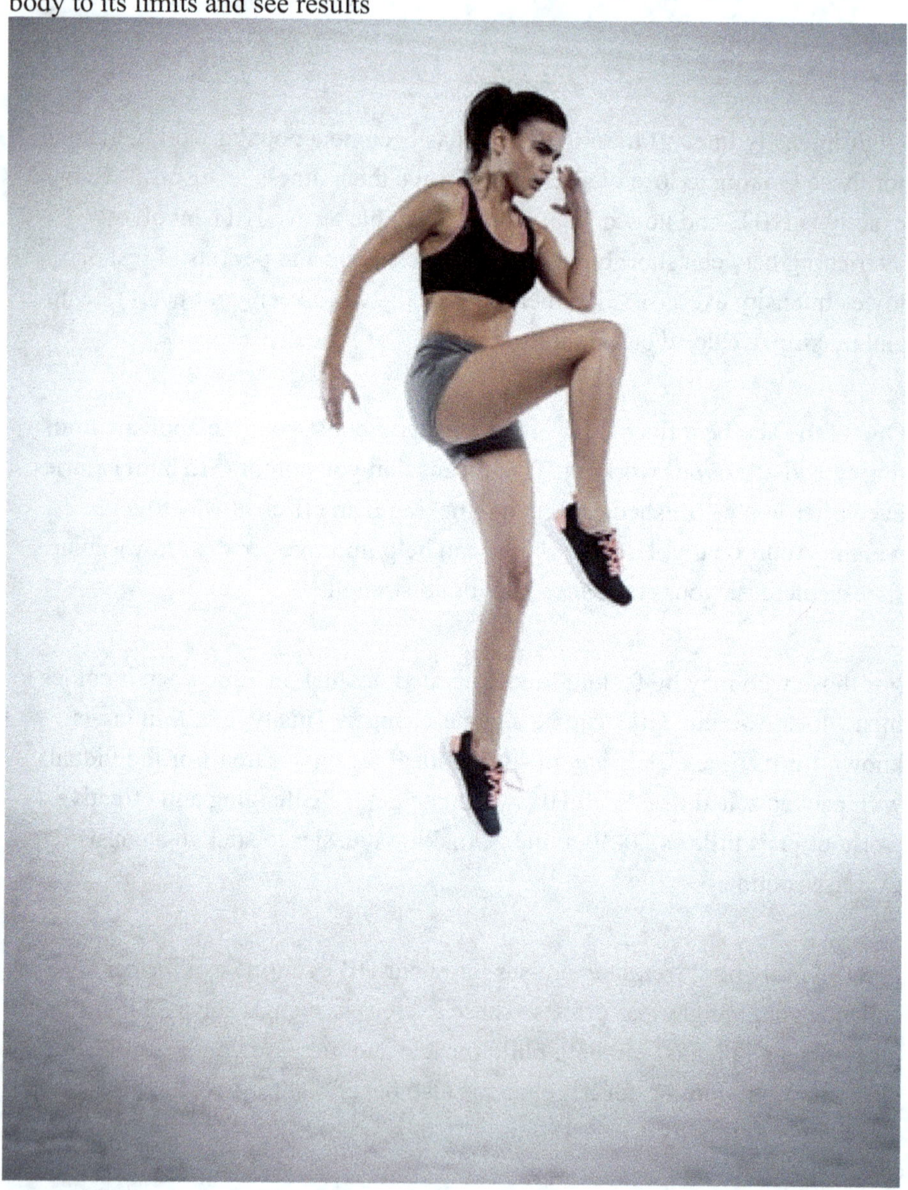

faster.

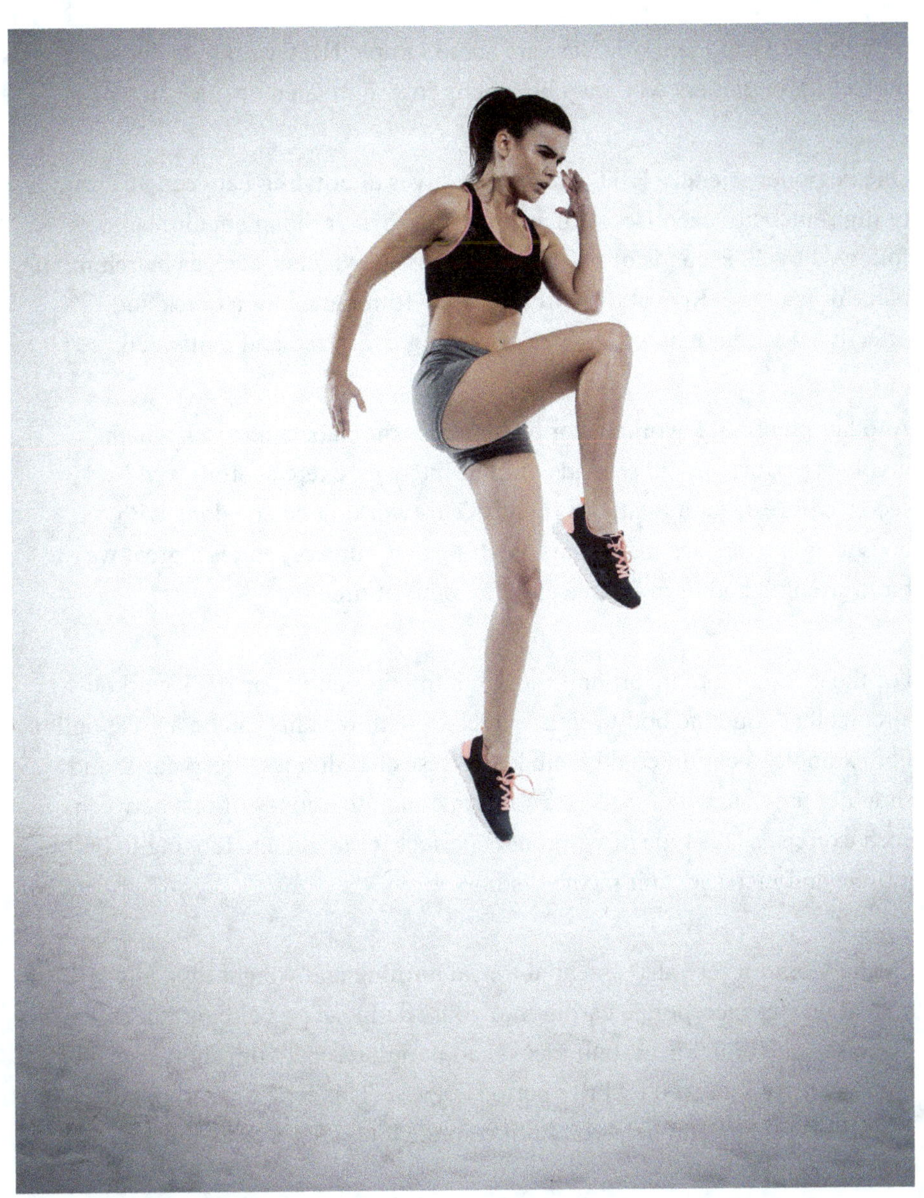

Sample HIIT Workouts for Beginners

High-intensity interval training (HIIT) workouts are a fantastic way for beginners to kickstart their weight loss journey and make lasting lifestyle changes. HIIT workouts are known for their efficiency and effectiveness in burning calories and fat, making them perfect for those looking to shed extra pounds and keep them off. Here are some sample HIIT workouts that are perfect for beginners who may be feeling low motivated or stuck in a rut.

One beginner-friendly HIIT workout involves alternating between 30 seconds of high-intensity exercise, such as jumping jacks or mountain climbers, followed by 30 seconds of rest or low-intensity exercise, such as marching in place or walking. Repeat this circuit for 10-15 minutes for a quick and effective workout that will leave you feeling energized and motivated.

Another great HIIT workout for beginners is the Tabata method, which involves performing 20 seconds of high-intensity exercise, followed by 10 seconds of rest, for a total of 8 rounds. This workout can be done with bodyweight exercises like squats, push-ups, or burpees, and is a great way to build strength and burn fat in a short amount of time.

For those looking to incorporate strength training into their HIIT workouts, circuits that combine bodyweight exercises with weights can be a great option. For example, a circuit could include exercises like lunges, bicep curls, and shoulder presses, with 30 seconds of work and 30 seconds of rest between each exercise. This type of workout is perfect for beginners looking to build muscle and increase their metabolism.

Cardio workouts are also essential for fat burning and weight loss, and HIIT is a great way to incorporate cardio into your routine. Try a circuit that includes exercises like high knees, butt kicks, and jumping rope, with short bursts of high intensity followed by brief periods of rest. This type of workout will get your heart rate up and help you burn calories long after you've finished exercising.

But perhaps my favorite is incorporating a simple yet effective HIIT workout into my routine by alternating between walking and running intervals. For example, I might start with a brisk walk for one minute to warm up, followed by a burst of running at a challenging pace for 30 seconds. After that, I'll return to a brisk walk for another minute to recover before repeating the cycle several times. This combination of walking and running intervals not only elevates my heart rate and boosts my metabolism but also allows me to maximize calorie burn and improve my cardiovascular fitness in a time-efficient manner.

In addition to these HIIT workouts, it's important to remember that nutrition plays a crucial role in weight loss and overall health. Meal planning and making healthy food choices are key components of a successful lifestyle change. By combining HIIT workouts with a balanced diet, you can achieve your weight loss goals and maintain a healthy lifestyle for years to come.

Advantages of HIIT for Weight Loss

High-intensity interval training (HIIT) has become increasingly popular in recent years, and for good reason. HIIT workouts are known for their effectiveness in burning calories and fat, making them an excellent choice for those looking to lose weight and keep it off. In this subchapter, we will explore the numerous advantages of HIIT for weight loss, particularly for individuals who may be feeling low motivated or stuck in a rut when it comes to their fitness journey.

One of the main advantages of HIIT for weight loss is its time efficiency. HIIT workouts typically involve short bursts of intense exercise followed by brief periods of rest or lower-intensity activity. This means that you can achieve the same (or even better) results in a fraction of the time compared to traditional steady-state cardio workouts. For busy Moms, Dads, or anyone struggling to find time for exercise, HIIT can be a game-changer.

Additionally, HIIT workouts have been shown to boost your metabolism, both during and after the workout. This is known as the "afterburn effect" or excess post-exercise oxygen consumption (EPOC), where your body continues to burn calories at an elevated rate even after you've finished exercising. This can help you to burn more calories throughout the day, even when you're not actively working out, making it easier to create a calorie deficit for weight loss.

Another advantage of HIIT for weight loss is its adaptability and scalability. HIIT workouts can be modified to suit individuals of all fitness levels, from beginners to advanced athletes. Whether you're new to exercise or looking to challenge yourself with more advanced movements, HIIT can be tailored to meet your needs and help you progress towards your weight loss goals.

Furthermore, HIIT workouts are highly effective for fat burning. By incorporating both cardio and strength training elements into one workout, HIIT can help you build lean muscle mass while simultaneously burning fat. This can lead to a more toned and defined physique, as well as improved overall body composition. For those looking to not only lose weight but also sculpt their bodies, HIIT can be a valuable tool in achieving their desired results.

In conclusion, HIIT offers numerous advantages for weight loss, making it a valuable tool for individuals looking to change their lifestyle and achieve lasting results. Whether you're a beginner just starting out on your fitness journey or someone who has been struggling to see progress, incorporating HIIT into your routine can help you break through plateaus and reach your weight loss goals. With its time efficiency, metabolism-boosting effects, adaptability, and fat-burning capabilities, HIIT has the potential to transform your body and your mindset towards a healthier, fitter lifestyle.

Chapter 4: Bodyweight Exercises for Weight Loss

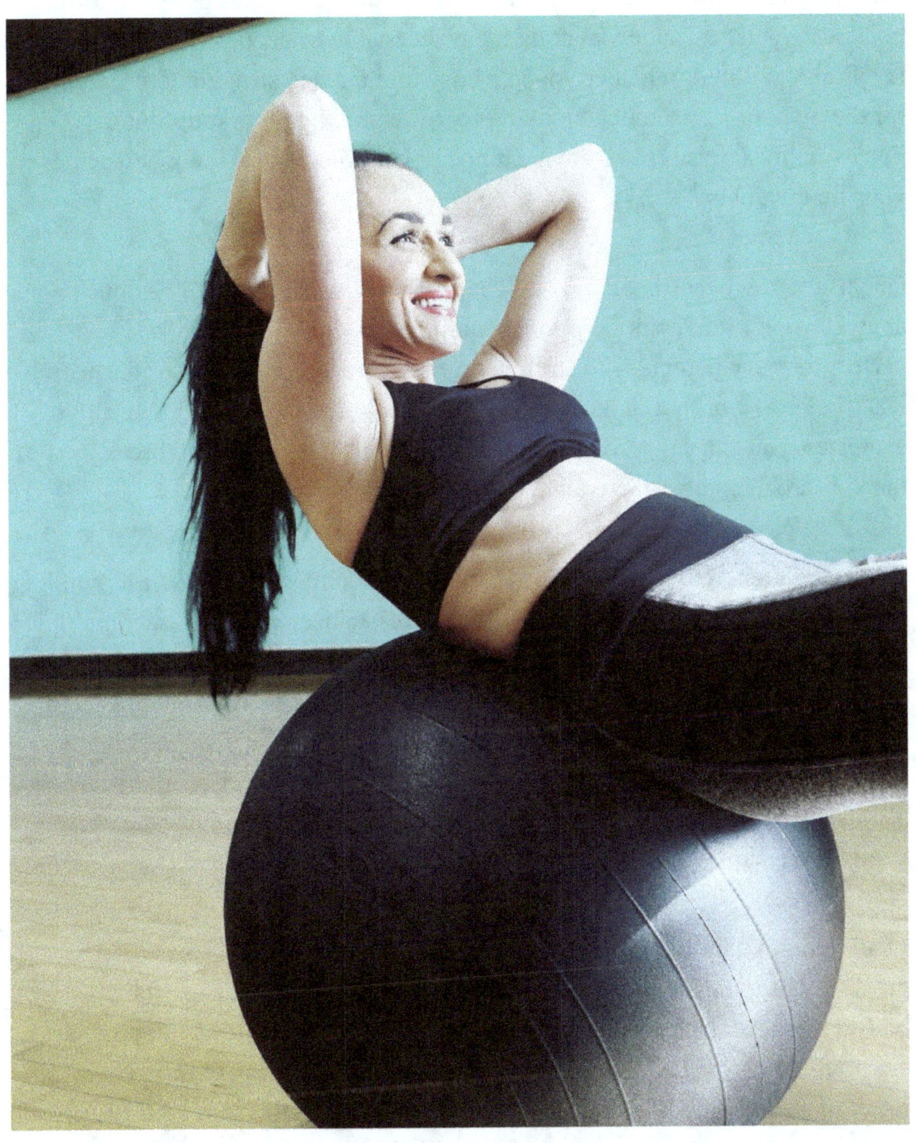

Benefits of Bodyweight Exercises

Bodyweight exercises are a fantastic way to kickstart your weight loss journey and improve your overall health and fitness. These exercises use your own body weight as resistance, making them accessible to people of all fitness levels and abilities. Whether you're a busy mom, a dad struggling to find time for the gym, or just someone looking to switch up their workout routine, bodyweight exercises offer a wide range of benefits that can help you achieve your fitness goals.

One of the key benefits of bodyweight exercises is that they can be done anywhere, anytime, with little to no equipment required. This makes them perfect for busy parents who struggle to find time to hit the gym or for people who prefer to workout in the comfort of their own home. With bodyweight exercises, you can squeeze in a quick workout during your lunch break, while the kids are napping, or even while watching TV in the evening.

Bodyweight exercises are also incredibly effective for weight loss and building muscle. By using your own body weight as resistance, you can target multiple muscle groups at once, leading to a more efficient and effective workout. Plus, bodyweight exercises can help increase your metabolism, burn calories, and improve your overall strength and endurance. Whether you're a beginner or a seasoned fitness enthusiast, incorporating bodyweight exercises into your routine can help you achieve your weight loss goals and build a leaner, stronger physique.

In addition to their weight loss benefits, bodyweight exercises also offer a great way to improve your cardiovascular fitness and endurance. Many bodyweight exercises, such as burpees, mountain climbers, and jumping jacks, are high-intensity interval training (HIIT) workouts that can elevate your heart rate and burn fat quickly. By incorporating these exercises into your routine, you can improve your cardiovascular health, boost your metabolism, and increase your overall fitness level.

Overall, bodyweight exercises offer a wide range of benefits for anyone looking to lose weight, build muscle, and improve their overall health and fitness. Whether you're a low-motivated parent, stuck in a rut, or just looking for a new workout challenge, incorporating bodyweight exercises into your routine can help you achieve your fitness goals and make lasting lifestyle changes. So, grab a yoga mat, clear some space in your living room, and get ready to sweat your way to a healthier, happier you with bodyweight exercises.

Sample Bodyweight Workouts for Weight Loss

In the quest to lose weight and keep it off, incorporating bodyweight workouts into your routine can be an effective and convenient way to achieve your fitness goals. Bodyweight exercises require no equipment and can be done anywhere, making them perfect for busy Moms, Dads, and anyone looking to make a lifestyle change. In this subchapter, we will explore some sample bodyweight workouts specifically designed for weight loss.

Bodyweight exercises for weight loss can help you build strength and increase muscle tone while burning calories. Examples of bodyweight exercises include squats, lunges, push-ups, and planks. These exercises can be modified to suit your fitness level and can be done at home or in a park. Strength training for beginners is a crucial component of any weight loss plan, as it helps to increase metabolism and build lean muscle mass.

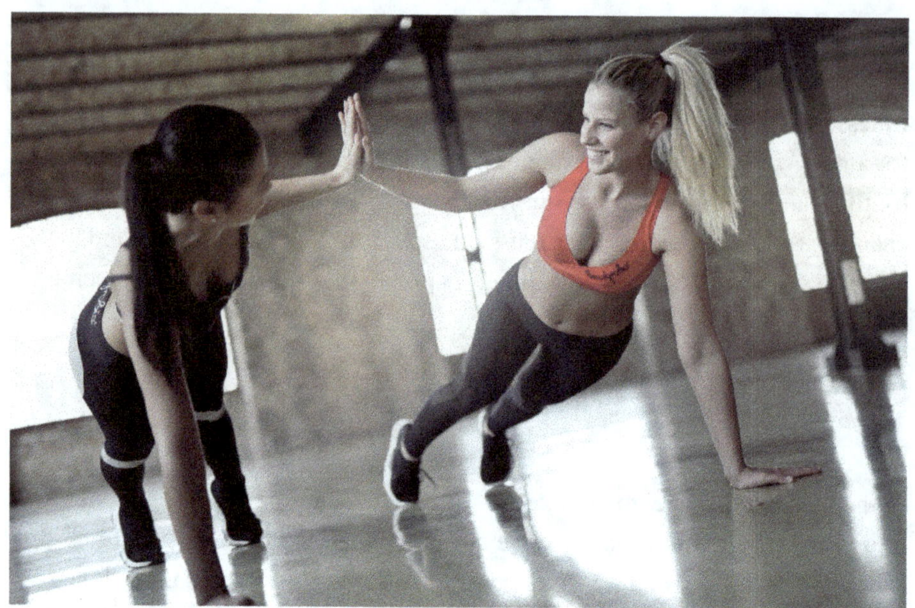

Cardio workouts for fat burning are essential for torching calories and improving cardiovascular health. Sample cardio workouts may include running or jogging, cycling, or jumping rope. These types of workouts can be done indoors or outdoors and can be tailored to your fitness level. Nutrition and meal planning for weight loss are also key factors in achieving your weight loss goals. Incorporating a balanced diet rich in fruits, vegetables, lean proteins, and whole grains can help fuel your body for workouts and promote weight loss.

In addition to bodyweight workouts, other forms of exercise such as yoga and Pilates can help improve flexibility, balance, and muscle tone. Weightlifting and muscle building exercises can also be beneficial for increasing metabolism and shaping your physique. Outdoor workouts for weight loss offer a refreshing change of scenery and can boost your mood and energy levels. By incorporating a variety of workouts into your routine and focusing on nutrition and meal planning, you can create a sustainable lifestyle change that supports your weight loss goals.

Progressing with Bodyweight Exercises

For those of you who are feeling stuck in a rut and struggling to find the motivation to lose weight and keep it off, incorporating bodyweight exercises into your fitness routine can be a game changer. Bodyweight exercises are a great way to build strength, improve flexibility, and burn calories without the need for any expensive equipment or gym memberships. Whether you're a busy mom, dad, or just someone looking to make a lifestyle change, bodyweight exercises can help you reach your weight loss goals.

One of the key benefits of bodyweight exercises is that they can be easily modified to suit your fitness level. If you're just starting out, you can begin with simple exercises like squats, lunges, and push-ups. As you progress and build strength, you can gradually increase the intensity by adding more repetitions or trying more advanced variations of the exercises. This progressive approach will not only help you see results faster, but it will also keep you motivated to continue pushing yourself.

I know when you first starting out exercising it can be discouraging if you can not do very many reps, but here is a guide to follow to help you increase your reps and build confidence while seeing tangible progress. While you can apply this to any bodyweight exercise lets you push ups as an example.

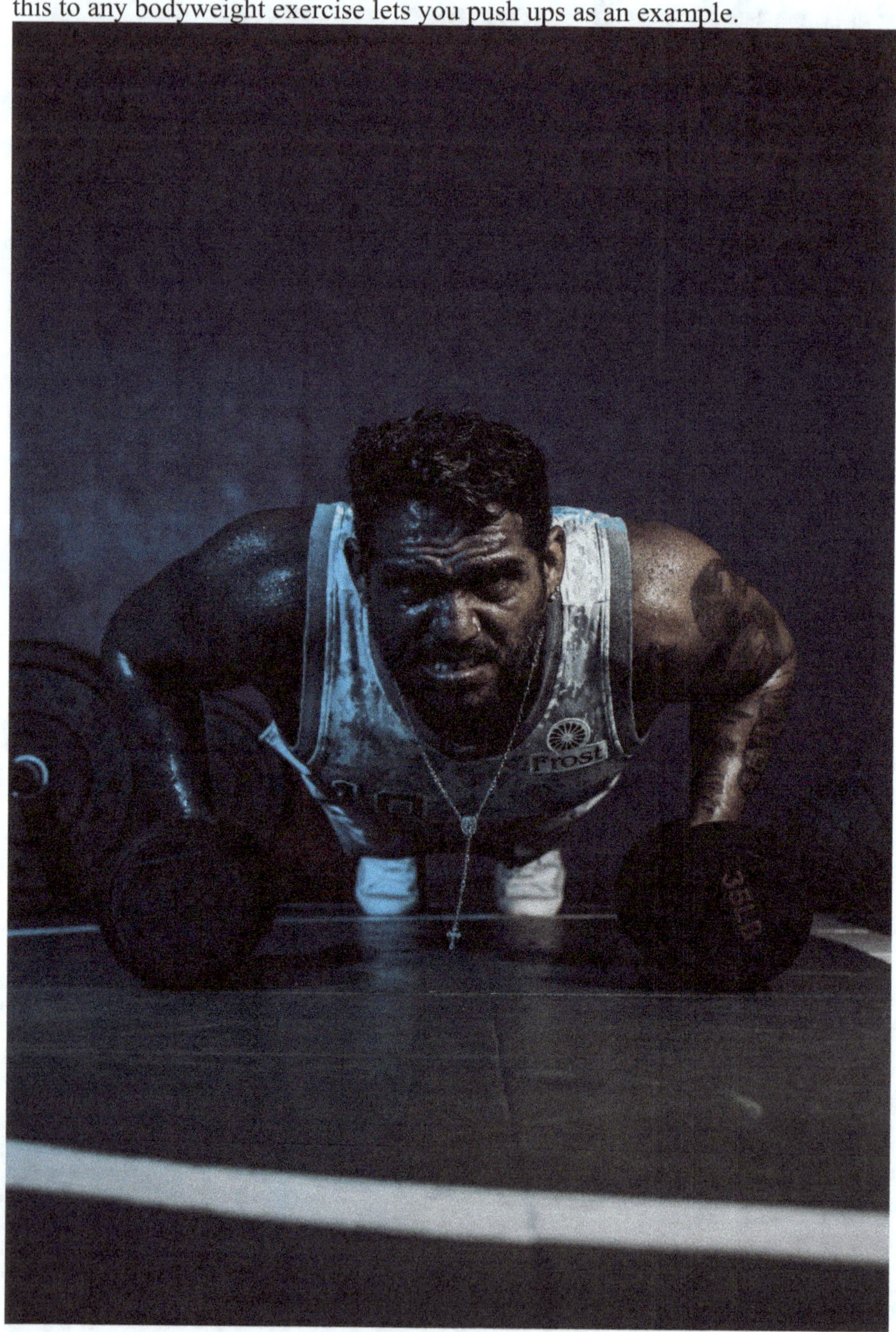

1. Practice Regularly: Consistent practice is key to improving your push-up strength. Set aside time to practice push-ups several times a week, gradually increasing the frequency and duration of your sessions.

2. Start with Modified Push-Ups: If regular push-ups are too challenging, start with modified versions such as knee push-ups or incline push-ups. These variations reduce the amount of body weight you have to lift, making them more manageable for beginners.

3. Focus on Proper Form: Pay attention to your form while performing push-ups to ensure maximum effectiveness and reduce the risk of injury. Keep your body in a straight line from head to heels, engage your core muscles, and lower yourself until your elbows reach a 90-degree angle before pushing back up.

4. Gradually Increase Reps: Start with a small number of push-ups that you can comfortably complete with good form, then gradually increase the number of repetitions as you build strength and endurance. Aim to add one or two more push-ups to each set every week.

5. Incorporate Strength Training: In addition to practicing push-ups, incorporate other strength training exercises that target the muscles used in push-ups, such as chest presses, triceps dips, and shoulder exercises. Building overall upper body strength will help you improve your push-up performance.

6. Rest and Recover: Allow your muscles adequate time to rest and recover between push-up sessions to prevent overtraining and promote muscle growth. Listen to your body and avoid pushing yourself too hard, especially if you're feeling fatigued or experiencing discomfort.

By following these tips and staying consistent with your training, you can gradually increase the number of push-ups you can do and improve your overall upper body strength.

High-intensity interval training (HIIT) workouts are another effective way to incorporate bodyweight exercises into your weight loss journey. This type of training has been shown to be highly effective for burning fat and improving cardiovascular fitness. By combining bodyweight exercises with HIIT, you can maximize your calorie burn and see results in a shorter amount of time.

Strength training for beginners can be intimidating, but bodyweight exercises provide a safe and effective way to build muscle and increase your overall strength. By focusing on exercises that target multiple muscle groups, such as planks, mountain climbers, and burpees, you can improve your muscular endurance and tone your body. As you become more comfortable with bodyweight exercises, you can gradually incorporate weights or resistance bands to further challenge your muscles and continue progressing towards your weight loss goals.

In addition to strength training, cardio workouts are essential for burning fat and improving your overall fitness level. Bodyweight exercises like jumping jacks, high knees, and mountain climbers are great for getting your heart rate up and torching calories. By incorporating a mix of bodyweight strength training and cardio exercises into your routine, you can create a well-rounded workout that will help you achieve your weight loss goals and maintain a healthy lifestyle. Remember, consistency is key when it comes to seeing results, so make sure to stay committed to your fitness routine and make healthy choices when it comes to nutrition and meal planning.

Chapter 5: Strength Training for Beginners

Importance of Strength Training for Weight Loss

Strength training is a crucial component of any weight loss journey, especially for those who are looking to not only shed pounds but also keep them off long-term. Many people mistakenly believe that cardio is the key to weight loss, but in reality, strength training plays a vital role in boosting metabolism and building lean muscle mass. By incorporating strength training into your workout routine, you can increase your overall calorie burn and improve your body composition.

One of the main reasons why strength training is so effective for weight loss is that it helps to increase muscle mass. Muscle tissue is more metabolically active than fat tissue, meaning that the more muscle you have, the more calories your body will burn at rest. This can help to speed up your metabolism and make it easier to maintain a healthy weight over time. Additionally, strength training can help to improve your overall strength and endurance, making it easier to perform everyday tasks and stay active.

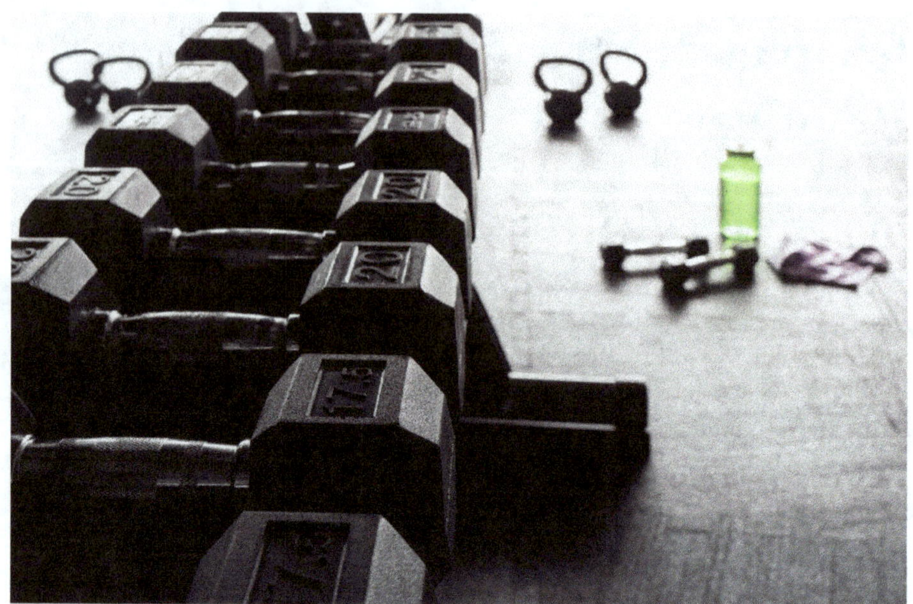

Another benefit of strength training for weight loss is that it can help to prevent muscle loss while you are in a calorie deficit. When you are trying to lose weight, your body may break down muscle tissue for energy if you are not providing it with enough fuel. By incorporating strength training into your routine, you can help to preserve lean muscle mass and ensure that the weight you are losing is coming from fat stores rather than muscle tissue.

In addition to its weight loss benefits, strength training can also help to improve your overall health and well-being. Regular strength training has been shown to reduce the risk of chronic diseases such as heart disease, diabetes, and osteoporosis. It can also help to improve your posture, balance, and coordination, making it easier to stay active and injury-free.

Overall, strength training is an essential component of any successful weight loss plan. By incorporating strength training into your workout routine, you can increase your metabolism, build lean muscle mass, and improve your overall health. Whether you are a beginner or have been working out for years, adding strength training to your routine can help you achieve your weight loss goals and maintain a healthy lifestyle for years to come.

Basic Strength Training Exercises for Beginners

Strength training is an essential component of any effective workout routine, especially for beginners looking to lose weight and keep it off. Basic strength training exercises are a great way to build muscle, increase metabolism, and improve overall fitness levels. For low motivated individuals who are stuck in a rut, incorporating these exercises into your routine can provide the motivation and momentum needed to make lasting lifestyle changes.

One of the simplest and most effective strength training exercises for beginners is the bodyweight squat. This exercise targets the muscles in the legs, glutes, and core, and can be easily modified to suit individual fitness levels. Start by standing with your feet shoulder-width apart, then lower your body by bending your knees and pushing your hips back. Make sure to keep your chest up and your back straight throughout the movement. Aim for 3 sets of 10-12 reps to start, gradually increasing the number of reps as your strength improves.

Another beginner-friendly strength training exercise is the bench press. This classic exercise works the muscles in the chest, shoulders, and triceps, while also engaging the core for added stability. To perform a proper bench press lie flat on a bench with your back, shoulders, and buttocks in contact with the bench. Your feet should be flat on the floor for stability.

Grip the barbell or dumbbells with your hands slightly wider than shoulder-width apart, palms facing forward. Lift the weight off the rack and hold it directly above your chest with your arms fully extended. This is the starting position. Lower the weight slowly and under control until it touches your chest, keeping your elbows at about a 90-degree angle. Push the weight back up to the starting position, extending your arms fully. Repeat for the desired number of repetitions, try and have a light enough weight to be able to do 10 - 12 reps.

It's important to use proper form while performing the bench press to prevent injury and maximize effectiveness. Keep your back flat against the bench, your feet firmly planted on the floor, and your elbows pointed slightly outward as you lower and raise the weight. Start with a weight that allows you to perform the exercise with good form, and gradually increase the weight as you become stronger.

For those looking to add some resistance to their strength training routine, dumbbell exercises are a great option. Dumbbells are versatile and can be used to target a wide range of muscle groups, making them ideal for beginners. Try incorporating exercises like bicep curls, shoulder presses, and bent-over rows into your workout to build strength and increase muscle tone. Start with a lighter weight and focus on proper form to prevent injury and maximize results.

Incorporating basic strength training exercises into your workout routine is a key step towards achieving your weight loss and fitness goals. By starting with simple exercises like squats, bench press, and dumbbell exercises, beginners can build a solid foundation of strength and muscle tone. Remember to listen to your body, start slowly, and gradually increase the intensity and difficulty of your workouts as you progress. With consistency and dedication, you can transform your body and create lasting lifestyle changes that will help you lose weight and keep it off for good.

Building Muscle to Boost Metabolism

Building muscle is an essential component of boosting metabolism and achieving long-term weight loss success. Many people believe that cardio is the key to burning fat and losing weight, but strength training is just as important, if not more so. When you build muscle, your body becomes more efficient at burning calories, even at rest. This means that you will continue to burn fat throughout the day, even when you're not actively working out.

One of the best ways to build muscle and boost metabolism is through high-intensity interval training (HIIT) workouts. These workouts involve short bursts of intense exercise followed by periods of rest or lower-intensity exercise. HIIT workouts are incredibly effective at burning fat and building muscle, making them a great choice for anyone looking to lose weight and keep it off. Plus, they can be done in a short amount of time, making them perfect for busy Moms, Dads, and anyone else with a hectic schedule.

Bodyweight exercises are another great option for building muscle and boosting metabolism, especially for beginners. These exercises, which use your own body weight as resistance, can be done anywhere, anytime, without the need for expensive equipment. Push-ups, squats, lunges, and planks are all examples of bodyweight exercises that can help you build muscle and burn fat. By incorporating these exercises into your routine, you can start to see real results in a short amount of time.

Strength training is also crucial for building muscle and boosting metabolism. Lifting weights or using resistance bands can help you build lean muscle mass, which in turn increases your metabolism and helps you burn more calories. Strength training can be intimidating for beginners, but with the right guidance and support, it can be a highly effective way to achieve your weight loss goals. Start with light weights and gradually increase the intensity as you become stronger and more confident in your abilities.

In addition to regular workouts, nutrition plays a key role in building muscle and boosting metabolism. Eating a balanced diet that includes plenty of protein, healthy fats, and complex carbohydrates will provide your body with the fuel it needs to build muscle and burn fat. Meal planning can help you stay on track with your nutrition goals and make healthy eating a habit. By combining regular workouts with a nutritious diet, you can create a lifestyle that supports your weight loss goals and helps you maintain your results in the long term.

Chapter 6: Cardio Workouts for Fat Burning

Understanding the Role of Cardio in Weight Loss

Understanding the role of cardio in weight loss is crucial for anyone looking to shed extra pounds and improve their overall health. Cardiovascular exercise, also known as cardio, is any type of physical activity that raises your heart rate and improves the efficiency of your heart and lungs. This type of exercise is essential for burning calories and fat, which can lead to weight loss when combined with a healthy diet.

For low motivated individuals, incorporating cardio into their daily routine can be a challenging task. However, it is important to remember that even small amounts of cardio can make a significant difference in weight loss. Starting with just 10-15 minutes of cardio a day, such as brisk walking or jumping jacks, can help kickstart your weight loss journey and increase your motivation to continue.

Stuck in a rut? Mixing up your cardio routine can help prevent boredom and keep you on track towards your weight loss goals. Try incorporating different types of cardio exercises, such as running, cycling, or swimming, to keep your workouts fresh and exciting. High-intensity interval training (HIIT) workouts are also a great way to maximize calorie burn and boost your metabolism.

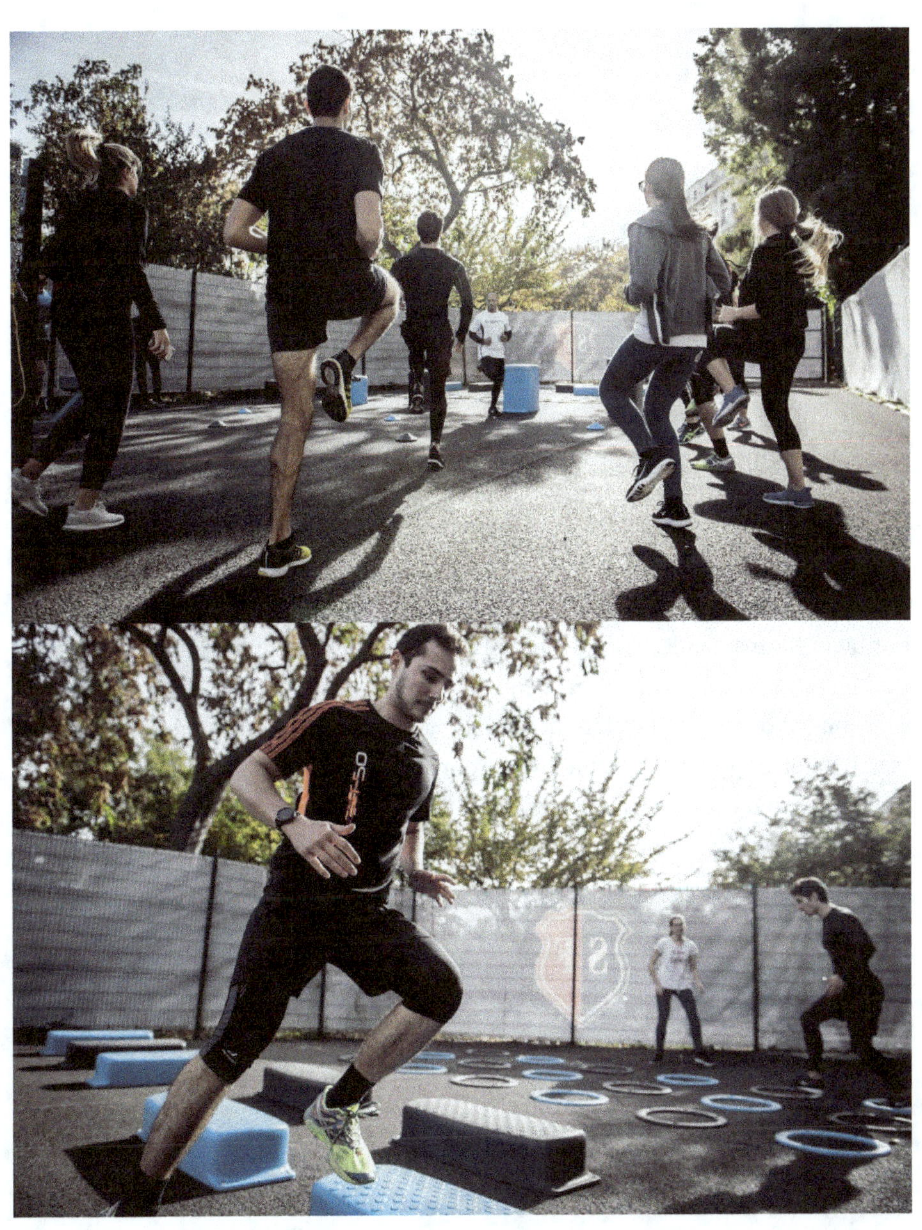

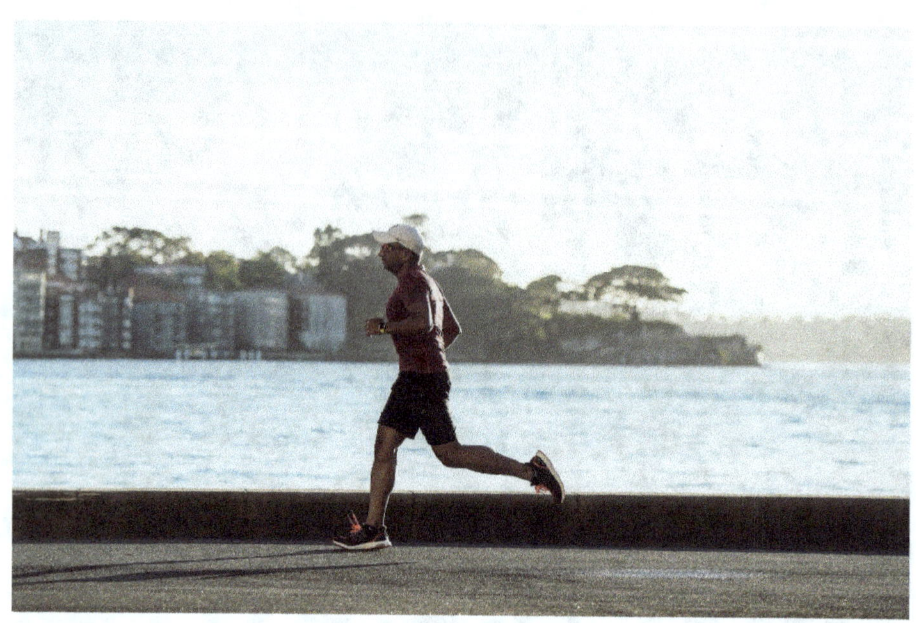

For busy Moms, Dads, and individuals looking to lose weight and keep it off, finding time for cardio workouts can be a challenge. However, incorporating short bursts of cardio throughout the day, such as taking the stairs instead of the elevator or going for a quick walk during your lunch break, can help you stay active and burn extra calories. Additionally, scheduling cardio sessions into your weekly routine can help you stay accountable and make exercise a priority.

In conclusion, understanding the role of cardio in weight loss is essential for anyone looking to make lasting lifestyle changes. By incorporating cardio into your daily routine, mixing up your workouts, and finding ways to stay active throughout the day, you can achieve your weight loss goals and improve your overall health. Remember, consistency is key, so stay motivated and stay

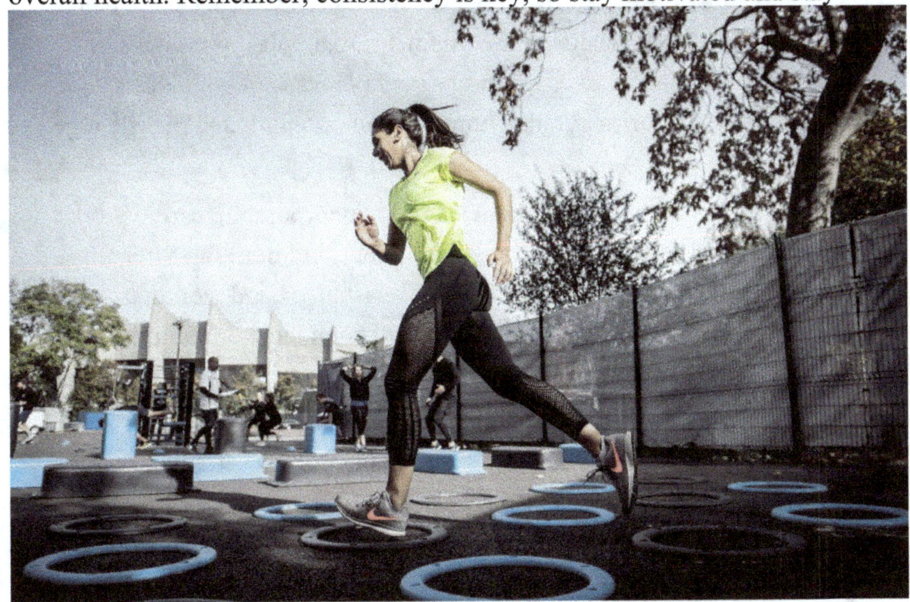

committed to your fitness journey.

Different Types of Cardio Workouts

When it comes to losing weight and keeping it off, incorporating cardio workouts into your routine is essential. Cardio exercises not only help you burn calories and fat, but they also improve your cardiovascular health and overall fitness level. There are many different types of cardio workouts to choose from, so you can find one that fits your preferences and fitness level.

One popular type of cardio workout is high-intensity interval training (HIIT). HIIT workouts involve short bursts of intense exercise followed by brief periods of rest or lower-intensity activity. This type of workout is great for burning calories quickly and improving your endurance. HIIT workouts can be done with bodyweight exercises, such as burpees, jumping jacks, and mountain climbers, making them a convenient option for those who prefer to exercise at home.

Bodyweight exercises are another effective form of cardio workout for weight loss. These exercises use your own body weight as resistance, so you can do them anywhere without the need for equipment. Examples of bodyweight exercises include squats, lunges, push-ups, and planks. These exercises not only help you burn calories but also improve your strength and muscle tone.

For beginners who are new to strength training, incorporating cardio workouts into your routine is a great way to build endurance and burn fat. Strength training exercises, such as weightlifting and resistance band workouts, can be combined with cardio exercises to create a well-rounded workout plan. Strength training helps you build muscle, which in turn boosts your metabolism and helps you burn more calories throughout the day.

If you're looking to specifically target fat burning, there are cardio workouts that are designed to maximize calorie burn and promote weight loss. These workouts typically involve exercises that elevate your heart rate and keep it elevated for an extended period of time, such as running, cycling, or jumping rope. These types of workouts are great for burning fat and improving your cardiovascular health.

No matter what type of cardio workout you choose, it's important to also focus on nutrition and meal planning for weight loss. Eating a balanced diet that includes plenty of fruits, vegetables, lean proteins, and whole grains will help support your fitness goals and fuel your workouts. Additionally, incorporating other forms of exercise, such as yoga and Pilates for toning and flexibility, or outdoor workouts for weight loss, can help keep your routine interesting and prevent boredom. Remember, consistency is key when it comes to making lifestyle changes, so find a cardio workout that you enjoy and stick with it to see long-lasting results.

Tips for Effective Fat Burning Cardio Workouts

For those who are looking to kickstart their weight loss journey and effectively burn fat through cardio workouts, here are some tips to help you get started. These tips are designed for low motivated individuals who may feel stuck in a rut and are seeking guidance on how to make lasting lifestyle changes.

First and foremost, it's important to find a cardio workout that you enjoy. Whether it's running, cycling, dancing, or swimming, choosing an activity that you look forward to will help keep you motivated and engaged. Remember, exercise should not feel like a chore – it should be something that brings you joy and makes you feel good about yourself.

High-intensity interval training (HIIT) workouts are a great option for those looking to burn fat quickly and efficiently. HIIT involves alternating between short bursts of intense exercise and brief periods of rest or lower-intensity activity. This type of workout has been shown to be highly effective for fat loss and can be done in a short amount of time, making it perfect for busy Moms, Dads, and individuals with hectic schedules.

Bodyweight exercises are another effective way to burn fat and build muscle. Exercises like squats, lunges, push-ups, and planks can be done anywhere, without the need for any equipment. These exercises not only help you burn calories during your workout, but they also increase your metabolism, allowing you to continue burning fat even after you've finished exercising.

Strength training is also an important component of any fat-burning workout routine. Building muscle helps increase your metabolism, making it easier to burn fat and maintain a healthy weight. For beginners, it's important to start with light weights and focus on proper form to prevent injury. As you become more comfortable with strength training, you can gradually increase the weight and intensity of your workouts.

In addition to cardio and strength training, it's important to pay attention to your nutrition and meal planning. Eating a balanced diet that is rich in fruits, vegetables, lean proteins, and whole grains will help fuel your workouts and support your weight loss goals. Planning your meals ahead of time and packing healthy snacks can help you avoid making impulsive food choices that may derail your progress. Remember, weight loss is not just about exercise – it's about making small, sustainable changes to your lifestyle that will help you achieve your goals in the long run.

Chapter 7: Nutrition and Meal Planning for Weight Loss

Importance of Nutrition in Weight Loss

Nutrition plays a crucial role in weight loss and overall health. Many people underestimate the importance of proper nutrition when trying to shed excess pounds. However, what you eat can make or break your weight loss journey. In fact, studies have shown that diet is even more important than exercise when it comes to losing weight and keeping it off. This is why it is essential to pay close attention to what you are putting into your body if you want to see real results.

When it comes to weight loss, the old saying "you are what you eat" could not be more true. The foods you consume on a daily basis have a direct impact on your energy levels, metabolism, and ability to burn fat. By focusing on a balanced diet rich in whole foods such as fruits, vegetables, lean proteins, and whole grains, you can fuel your body with the nutrients it needs to function optimally. On the other hand, processed foods high in sugar, sodium, and unhealthy fats can sabotage your weight loss efforts and leave you feeling sluggish and unmotivated.

In addition to providing your body with the right nutrients, proper nutrition can also help you control your appetite and cravings. When you eat a diet high in fiber, protein, and healthy fats, you are more likely to feel full and satisfied after meals, reducing the likelihood of overeating or snacking on unhealthy foods. By choosing nutrient-dense options and practicing portion control, you can keep your hunger in check and stay on track with your weight loss goals.

Furthermore, nutrition plays a key role in supporting your body through exercise and physical activity. Whether you are engaging in high-intensity interval training, strength training, or cardio workouts, your body needs the right fuel to perform at its best. By eating a balanced diet that includes a mix of carbohydrates, proteins, and fats, you can optimize your energy levels and recover more quickly from intense workouts. This will not only help you see better results in the gym but also improve your overall health and well-being.

Overall, the importance of nutrition in weight loss cannot be overstated. By making smart food choices and prioritizing a balanced diet, you can set yourself up for success on your weight loss journey. Remember, it's not just about cutting calories or following the latest fad diet – it's about nourishing your body with the nutrients it needs to thrive. With a focus on nutrition, you can achieve your weight loss goals, improve your health, and create lasting lifestyle changes that will benefit you for years to come.

Different Types of Diets for Weight Loss

When it comes to weight loss, there are a multitude of diets to choose from. However, not all diets are created equal, and it's important to find one that works best for you and your lifestyle. In this subchapter, we will explore different types of diets for weight loss that can help you reach your goals and maintain a healthy lifestyle.

One popular diet for weight loss is the ketogenic diet, which focuses on consuming high amounts of healthy fats, moderate protein, and very low carbohydrates. This diet aims to put the body into a state of ketosis, where it burns fat for fuel instead of carbohydrates. While this diet can be effective for some individuals, it may not be sustainable or practical for everyone.

So lets talk pros and cons of the keto type of diet.
Pros:
 Rapid Weight Loss: The ketogenic diet is known for its ability to promote rapid weight loss, particularly in the initial stages. By drastically reducing carbohydrate intake and increasing fat consumption, the body enters a state of ketosis, where it burns stored fat for fuel instead of glucose.

Appetite Control: The high-fat, moderate-protein nature of the keto diet can help regulate appetite and reduce cravings, making it easier to adhere to a calorie-restricted eating plan.

Improved Blood Sugar Control: Some research suggests that the keto diet may help improve insulin sensitivity and blood sugar control, which can be beneficial for individuals with type 2 diabetes or prediabetes.

Increased Energy Levels: Once adapted to using ketones as a primary fuel source, many people report experiencing sustained energy levels throughout the day without the energy crashes associated with carb-heavy diets.

Mental Clarity and Focus: Some individuals on the keto diet report experiencing improved mental clarity, concentration, and cognitive function, which may be attributed to stable blood sugar levels and ketone metabolism.

Cons:
Initial Side Effects: Many people experience "keto flu" symptoms in the first few days or weeks of starting the diet, including fatigue, headaches, dizziness, nausea, and irritability. These side effects typically subside as the body adjusts to ketosis.

Restrictive Nature: The keto diet requires strict adherence to macronutrient ratios, with a significant reduction in carbohydrate intake and a higher emphasis on fat consumption. This can be challenging for some individuals to maintain long-term, especially in social situations or when dining out.

Potential Nutrient Deficiencies: Because the keto diet restricts many food groups rich in essential nutrients, such as fruits, whole grains, and legumes, there is a risk of nutrient deficiencies if the diet is not properly planned. It's essential to focus on nutrient-dense foods and consider supplementation as needed.
Digestive Issues: Some individuals may experience digestive issues such as constipation, diarrhea, or gastrointestinal discomfort when transitioning to a

high-fat, low-fiber diet. Increasing fiber intake from non-starchy vegetables and incorporating sources of healthy fats can help alleviate these symptoms.
Long-Term Health Effects: While short-term studies suggest potential benefits of the keto diet for weight loss and metabolic health, the long-term effects of sustained ketosis on overall health are still not well understood. Some concerns have been raised about the impact of high-fat intake on cardiovascular health, kidney function, and gut microbiota composition.

Ultimately, whether the keto diet is suitable for an individual depends on various factors, including their health status, personal preferences, and lifestyle considerations. It's essential to consult with a healthcare professional or registered dietitian before making significant dietary changes to ensure they are safe and appropriate for your individual needs.

Another option is the Mediterranean diet, which emphasizes whole foods such as fruits, vegetables, whole grains, and healthy fats like olive oil and nuts. This diet is not only effective for weight loss, but it is also known for its heart-healthy benefits and ability to reduce the risk of chronic diseases such as diabetes and hypertension.

Now lets dive into the pros and cons of the Mediterranean diet.
Pros:
Heart Health Benefits: The Mediterranean diet is associated with numerous heart-healthy benefits, including reduced risk of heart disease, lower cholesterol levels, and improved blood pressure control. This is attributed to the emphasis on heart-healthy fats from sources such as olive oil, nuts, and fatty fish, as well as a high intake of fruits, vegetables, whole grains, and legumes. Rich in

Nutrients: The Mediterranean diet emphasizes nutrient-dense foods such as fruits, vegetables, whole grains, nuts, seeds, and lean proteins. This provides a wide range of essential vitamins, minerals, antioxidants, and phytonutrients that support overall health and well-being.

Sustainable and Flexible: Unlike many restrictive diets, the Mediterranean diet is flexible and adaptable to individual preferences and cultural traditions. It encourages a balanced approach to eating, allowing for a variety of foods and occasional indulgences while promoting long-term sustainability and enjoyment.

Weight Management: Research suggests that the Mediterranean diet may be effective for weight management and weight loss when combined with calorie control and regular physical activity. The high fiber content, moderate protein intake, and emphasis on whole, minimally processed foods help promote satiety and reduce overeating.

Delicious and Enjoyable: One of the key attractions of the Mediterranean diet is its delicious and flavorful cuisine. With its emphasis on fresh, seasonal ingredients, herbs, spices, and healthy fats, the Mediterranean diet offers a wide range of delicious and satisfying meals that can be enjoyed by the whole family.
Cons:

Potential Cost: While the Mediterranean diet emphasizes whole, minimally processed foods, some of the key components such as olive oil, nuts, and seafood can be expensive compared to other dietary patterns. This may make it less accessible to individuals on a tight budget.

Requires Cooking Skills: Many of the traditional foods and recipes associated with the Mediterranean diet require basic cooking skills and preparation time. For individuals with limited time or culinary expertise, following the Mediterranean diet may be challenging. Reliance on Fresh

Ingredients: The Mediterranean diet emphasizes fresh, seasonal ingredients, which may not be readily available or affordable for everyone, especially in certain geographic regions or during certain times of the year. This could pose challenges for individuals with limited access to fresh produce or limited transportation options.

Potential for Overconsumption: While the Mediterranean diet is rich in nutrient-dense foods, it can still be high in calories if portions are not controlled. Certain components of the diet, such as nuts, olive oil, and cheese, are calorie-dense and should be consumed in moderation to avoid excess calorie intake. Cultural and Social Considerations: The Mediterranean diet is deeply rooted in the culinary traditions and cultural practices of Mediterranean countries.

For individuals from different cultural backgrounds or dietary preferences, adopting the Mediterranean diet may require adjustments and compromises. Additionally, social occasions and dining out may present challenges for adhering to the principles of the Mediterranean diet.

Overall, the Mediterranean diet offers numerous health benefits and delicious culinary options, but it's important to consider individual preferences, resources, and cultural factors when deciding whether it's the right dietary approach for you. Consulting with a healthcare professional or registered dietitian can help tailor the Mediterranean diet to your specific needs and goals.

Intermittent fasting is another popular approach to weight loss that involves cycling between periods of eating and fasting. This can help regulate hormones, improve metabolism, and promote fat loss. There are several different methods of intermittent fasting, so it's important to find one that fits your lifestyle and goals.

Now this is my personal favorite. I have used this to control my eating and weight gain for years. Lets take a look at some different kind of intermittent fasting and the pros and cons of them as well.

1. 16/8 Method (also known as the Leangains protocol):
Pros:
Simplistic approach: Involves fasting for 16 hours each day and limiting eating to an 8-hour window.

Easy to implement: Requires minimal tracking and can fit into most daily schedules.

Potential for weight loss: Restricting eating to a shorter window may lead to reduced calorie intake and weight loss.

Cons:
Requires discipline: Some individuals may find it challenging to abstain from food for 16 hours.

Potential for overeating: There may be a tendency to overconsume calories during the eating window, negating potential weight loss benefits.

2. 5:2 Diet:
Pros:

Flexible: Involves eating normally for five days of the week and restricting calorie intake to 500-600 calories on two non-consecutive days.

Potential health benefits: May promote weight loss, improve metabolic health, and reduce the risk of chronic diseases.

Easy to adhere to: Offers flexibility in choosing fasting days based on individual preferences and schedules.

Cons:

Hunger and fatigue: Some individuals may experience hunger, fatigue, and irritability on fasting days, especially in the initial stages.

Potential for overconsumption: There may be a tendency to overeat on non-fasting days, which can hinder weight loss efforts.

Requires planning: Planning low-calorie meals for fasting days and ensuring adequate nutrition on non-fasting days may require effort and preparation.

3. Eat-Stop-Eat:

Pros:

Simple and straightforward: Involves fasting for 24 hours once or twice a week.

Potential for weight loss: Extended fasting periods may lead to reduced calorie intake and promote fat loss.

Improved insulin sensitivity: May help improve insulin sensitivity and blood sugar control.

Cons:

Hunger and discomfort: Extended fasting periods may lead to feelings of hunger, fatigue, and discomfort.

Potential for nutrient deficiencies: Prolonged fasting may increase the risk of nutrient deficiencies if not carefully planned and balanced.

Not suitable for everyone: Extended fasting may not be suitable for individuals with certain medical conditions or dietary restrictions.

4. Alternate-Day Fasting:

Pros:

Structured approach: Involves alternating between fasting days and non-fasting days.

Potential for weight loss: Alternate-day fasting may lead to reduced calorie intake and promote weight loss.

Simplifies meal planning: Eliminates the need for calorie counting or portion control on fasting days.

Cons:

Hunger and cravings: Some individuals may experience intense hunger and cravings on fasting days, which can be challenging to manage.

Disruption of social life: Alternate-day fasting may interfere with social activities and mealtime traditions, making it difficult to adhere to in social settings.

Potential for binge eating: There may be a tendency to overeat on non-fasting days, especially if food restriction is perceived as deprivation.

It's essential to consider individual preferences, lifestyle factors, and health status when choosing an intermittent fasting protocol. Consulting with a healthcare professional or registered dietitian can help determine the most appropriate approach and ensure safety and effectiveness.

The plant-based diet is another option for weight loss that focuses on consuming whole, plant-based foods such as fruits, vegetables, legumes, and grains. This diet is not only beneficial for weight loss, but it is also environmentally friendly and can reduce the risk of chronic diseases.

Alright lets expand on the plant-based diet with another pros and cons.

Pros:

Health Benefits:

Lower risk of chronic diseases: A plant-based diet rich in fruits, vegetables, whole grains, legumes, nuts, and seeds is associated with a reduced risk of heart disease, stroke, type 2 diabetes, certain cancers, and other chronic conditions.

Weight management: Plant-based diets are generally lower in calories and saturated fats while being higher in fiber, which can aid in weight management and promote satiety.

Improved overall health: Plant-based diets are often rich in vitamins, minerals, antioxidants, and phytonutrients, which support overall health, immune function, and longevity.

Environmental Sustainability: Reduced carbon footprint: Plant-based diets require fewer natural resources, land, water, and energy compared to animal-based diets, making them more environmentally sustainable and reducing greenhouse gas emissions.

Preservation of biodiversity: By reducing the demand for animal agriculture, plant-based diets help conserve biodiversity and protect ecosystems, including forests, wetlands, and wildlife habitats.

Ethical Considerations:

Animal welfare: Plant-based diets align with ethical considerations by reducing the demand for animal products and minimizing the suffering of animals raised for food production.

Compassion and empathy: Choosing plant-based foods promotes compassion and empathy towards animals and fosters a more sustainable and compassionate food system.

Variety and Flavor: Culinary diversity: Plant-based diets offer a wide variety of flavors, textures, and cuisines from around the world, allowing for creativity and exploration in the kitchen.

Access to seasonal and local produce: Plant-based diets encourage the consumption of seasonal, local, and fresh produce, supporting local farmers and promoting food diversity.

Cons:

Nutritional Considerations:

Potential nutrient deficiencies: Plant-based diets may be deficient in certain nutrients, including vitamin B12, iron, calcium, omega-3 fatty acids, and protein, if not properly planned and balanced.

Risk of processed foods: Plant-based diets may include highly processed and refined foods, such as vegan desserts, snacks, and convenience foods, which can be high in added sugars, sodium, and unhealthy fats.

Social and Cultural Challenges:

Limited dining options: Plant-based eaters may face challenges when dining out or attending social gatherings where plant-based options are limited or unavailable, leading to feelings of exclusion or inconvenience.

Cultural traditions and norms: Plant-based diets may conflict with cultural traditions, dietary preferences, and family customs, making it difficult for some individuals to adhere to or adopt.

Perceived Cost and Accessibility:

Perceived cost: Some people may perceive plant-based diets as more expensive due to the higher cost of organic produce, specialty plant-based products, and vegan alternatives.

Accessibility: Access to fresh, affordable, and diverse plant-based foods may be limited in certain geographic regions, rural areas, or low-income communities, leading to disparities in food access and availability.

Potential Social Stigma:

Social stigma and judgment: Plant-based eaters may encounter social stigma, criticism, or judgment from friends, family members, or colleagues who may hold negative stereotypes or misconceptions about plant-based diets.

Misinformation and skepticism: Plant-based diets may be met with skepticism or skepticism from individuals who believe that animal products are essential for health or view plant-based eating as extreme or unconventional.

Overall, the decision to adopt a plant-based diet should be based on individual preferences, health considerations, ethical beliefs, and cultural factors. It's essential to approach plant-based eating with balance, mindfulness, and consideration for nutritional adequacy to ensure long-term health and well-being. Consulting with a healthcare professional or registered dietitian can provide personalized guidance and support in adopting a plant-based diet that meets individual needs and goals.

Regardless of the diet you choose, it's important to focus on making sustainable lifestyle changes that you can maintain in the long term. It's also important to consult with a healthcare professional or registered dietitian before starting any new diet to ensure it is safe and effective for you. By finding a diet that works for you and incorporating regular exercise and healthy habits, you can achieve your weight loss goals and maintain a healthy lifestyle for years to come.

Creating a Healthy Meal Plan for Weight Loss

One of the most important aspects of losing weight and keeping it off is creating a healthy meal plan. This is especially true for busy parents and individuals who may feel stuck in a rut when it comes to their eating habits. By taking the time to plan out your meals in advance, you can ensure that you are getting the nutrients you need while also controlling your calorie intake.

When creating a healthy meal plan for weight loss, it's important to focus on whole, unprocessed foods. This means incorporating plenty of fruits, vegetables, lean proteins, and whole grains into your diet. These foods are not only nutrient-dense, but they are also lower in calories than processed foods, which can help you achieve your weight loss goals.

In addition to focusing on whole foods, it's also important to pay attention to portion sizes when creating your meal plan. Many people underestimate the amount of food they are actually eating, which can lead to consuming more calories than necessary. By measuring out your portions and being mindful of serving sizes, you can better control your calorie intake and support your weight loss efforts.

Another key component of a healthy meal plan for weight loss is balance. This means incorporating a mix of carbohydrates, proteins, and fats into each meal. Carbohydrates provide energy, proteins support muscle growth and repair, and fats help with satiety and nutrient absorption. By including all three macronutrients in each meal, you can ensure that you are getting a well-rounded diet that supports your weight loss goals.

Finally, it's important to remember that a healthy meal plan is just one piece of the puzzle when it comes to losing weight and keeping it off. It's also important to stay active, whether through high-intensity interval training, bodyweight exercises, strength training, cardio workouts, yoga, or Pilates. By combining a healthy meal plan with regular exercise, you can maximize your weight loss results and create a sustainable lifestyle change that supports your overall health and well-being.

Tips for Eating Out While Trying to Lose Weight

Eating out can be a challenge when you're trying to lose weight, but with some planning and smart choices, you can still enjoy dining out while staying on track with your weight loss goals. Here are some tips to help you navigate restaurant menus and make healthier choices when eating out.

First and foremost, it's important to do some research before heading out to eat. Many restaurants now provide their menus and nutritional information online, so take advantage of this and plan out what you're going to order ahead of time. Look for options that are lower in calories, saturated fats, and sugars, and opt for dishes that are grilled, baked, or steamed rather than fried.

When you arrive at the restaurant, don't be afraid to ask your server for modifications to your meal. Most restaurants are more than happy to accommodate special requests, such as dressing on the side, substituting vegetables for fries, or asking for a smaller portion size. By customizing your meal to fit your dietary needs, you can enjoy dining out without derailing your weight loss progress.

Another tip for eating out while trying to lose weight is to practice mindful eating. Take your time to savor each bite, chew slowly, and pay attention to your hunger cues. Stop eating when you're full, even if there's still food on your plate. Remember, you don't have to clean your plate – it's okay to leave food behind if you're satisfied.

Choosing healthier options doesn't mean you have to sacrifice flavor. Look for dishes that are packed with vegetables, lean proteins, and whole grains, and don't be afraid to experiment with new flavors and cuisines. Many restaurants offer delicious and nutritious options that can help you stay on track with your weight loss goals while still enjoying a satisfying meal.

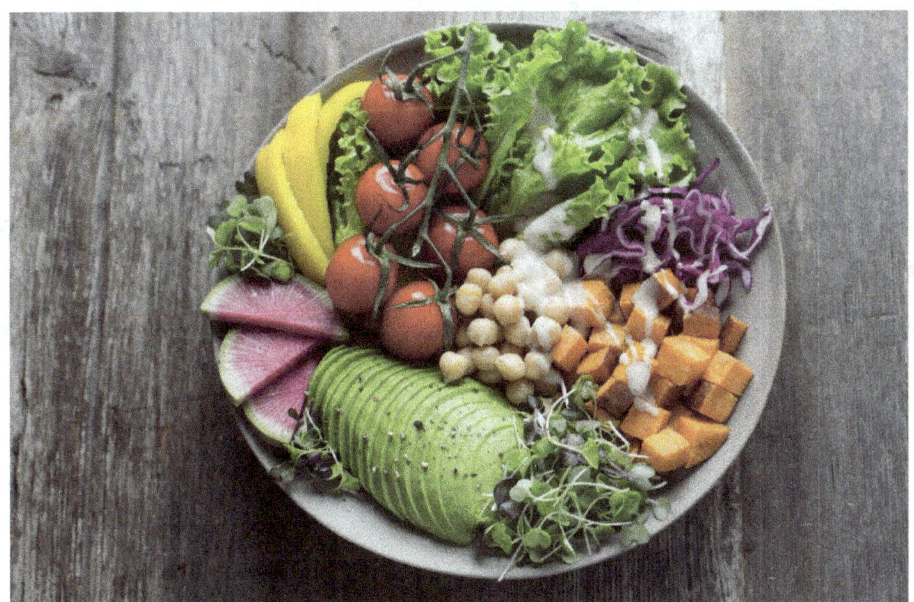

Lastly, don't be too hard on yourself if you indulge in a treat or two while eating out. It's important to practice balance and moderation, so if you have a dessert or high-calorie meal, simply make healthier choices for your next meal or snack. Remember, weight loss is a journey, and it's all about progress, not perfection. By following these tips and making smart choices when eating out, you can stay on track with your weight loss goals and enjoy dining out with friends and family.

Chapter 8: Yoga and Pilates for Toning and Flexibility

Benefits of Yoga and Pilates for Weight Loss

Yoga and Pilates are not only great for toning and flexibility, but they can also be incredibly effective tools for weight loss. These mind-body practices offer a holistic approach to fitness that can help you shed pounds and keep them off in the long run. By incorporating Yoga and Pilates into your routine, you can reap a wide range of benefits that go beyond just physical weight loss.

One of the key benefits of Yoga and Pilates for weight loss is their ability to increase muscle tone and strength. Both practices involve a series of movements and poses that engage and challenge your muscles, leading to improved muscle definition and a higher metabolism. This can help you burn more calories throughout the day, even when you're not actively working out. Additionally, building lean muscle mass can help boost your overall energy levels and increase your endurance, making it easier to stick to your weight loss goals.

Another advantage of Yoga and Pilates for weight loss is their focus on mindfulness and stress reduction. Both practices emphasize deep breathing, relaxation, and mental focus, which can help reduce cortisol levels and lower stress levels. High stress levels have been linked to weight gain and difficulty losing weight, so incorporating Yoga and Pilates into your routine can help you manage stress and improve your overall well-being. By taking time to care for your mental and emotional health, you can create a more sustainable and effective approach to weight loss.

Yoga and Pilates also offer a low-impact alternative to traditional cardio workouts, making them ideal for individuals who may have joint pain or other physical limitations. These practices can help improve your balance, coordination, and flexibility, while also providing a gentle yet effective cardiovascular workout. By incorporating Yoga and Pilates into your routine, you can strengthen your body without putting unnecessary strain on your joints, making it easier to stick to your weight loss goals in the long term.

In addition to their physical benefits, Yoga and Pilates can also help improve your overall body awareness and posture. By focusing on alignment, breathing, and core strength, these practices can help you develop a stronger, more stable foundation for all of your movements. This can help prevent injuries and improve your overall athletic performance, making it easier to stay active and engaged in your weight loss journey. By prioritizing proper form and alignment in your Yoga and Pilates practice, you can build a strong and balanced body that supports your weight loss goals.

Overall, Yoga and Pilates offer a comprehensive and holistic approach to weight loss that can benefit individuals of all fitness levels. By incorporating these practices into your routine, you can improve your muscle tone, reduce stress, and increase your overall body awareness and posture. Whether you're a beginner looking to kickstart your weight loss journey or a seasoned athlete looking to mix up your routine, Yoga and Pilates can offer a wide range of benefits that can help you achieve your goals and maintain a healthy lifestyle for years to come.

Sample Yoga and Pilates Workouts for Beginners

Incorporating yoga and Pilates into your workout routine can be a great way to enhance flexibility, improve strength, and relieve stress. These low-impact exercises are perfect for beginners who may be looking for a gentle introduction to fitness. In this subchapter, we will explore some sample yoga and Pilates workouts that are tailored specifically for those who are new to these practices.

One of the key benefits of yoga and Pilates is their ability to improve flexibility. For beginners, it's important to start with simple poses and movements that focus on stretching and lengthening the muscles. A sample yoga workout may include poses like child's pose, downward facing dog, and warrior one. These poses can help to increase flexibility in the hips, hamstrings, and back, while also promoting relaxation and stress relief.

Pilates, on the other hand, focuses on core strength and stability. A sample Pilates workout for beginners may include exercises like the hundred, leg circles, and the plank. These exercises can help to strengthen the abdominal muscles, improve posture, and enhance overall body awareness. Pilates is also known for its ability to improve balance and coordination, making it a great addition to any fitness routine.

For those who are looking to lose weight and keep it off, incorporating yoga and Pilates into their workout routine can be a game-changer. These practices not only help to improve physical fitness, but they also promote mental well-being and mindfulness. By combining these exercises with a healthy diet and lifestyle changes, individuals can achieve long-lasting weight loss results.

Whether you're a busy mom, a dad stuck in a rut, or simply someone looking to make a lifestyle change, yoga and Pilates can be the perfect addition to your fitness routine. These gentle yet effective exercises can help you build strength, improve flexibility, and reduce stress. So why not give it a try and see the amazing benefits for yourself? Remember, it's never too late to start on the path to a healthier, happier you.

Improving Flexibility and Strength through Yoga and Pilates

Improving flexibility and strength through yoga and Pilates can be a game-changer for those looking to lose weight and keep it off. These low-impact exercises not only tone and strengthen muscles, but they also improve flexibility, posture, and overall well-being. For busy moms, dads, and individuals stuck in a rut, incorporating yoga and Pilates into their fitness routine can provide a much-needed escape from the stresses of everyday life.

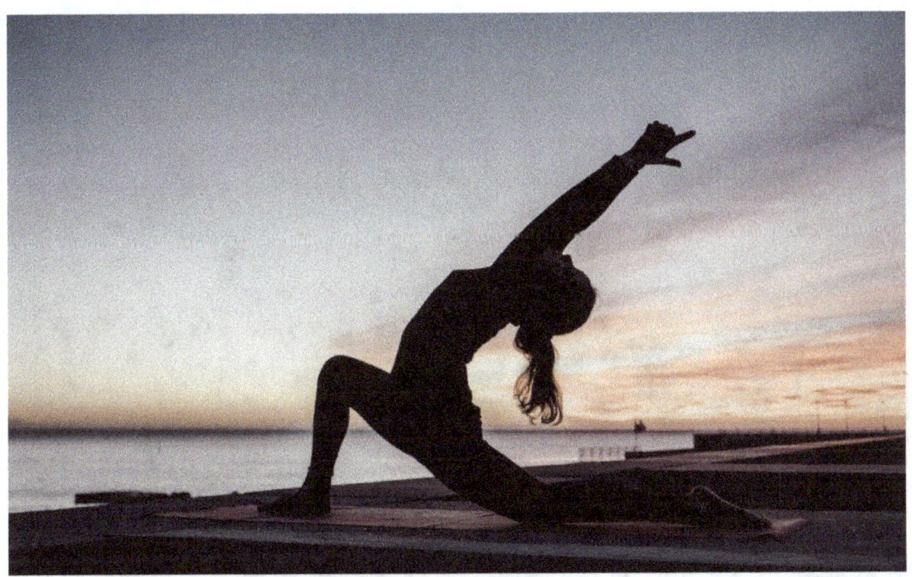

Yoga and Pilates are both excellent forms of exercise for beginners and those looking to ease into a workout routine. These practices focus on controlled movements, breathing techniques, and mindfulness, making them ideal for individuals who may be intimidated by more high-intensity workouts. By starting with yoga and Pilates, individuals can gradually build strength and flexibility, eventually leading to more challenging workouts and greater weight loss results.

One of the key benefits of yoga and Pilates is their ability to target specific muscle groups, helping individuals tone and sculpt their bodies. Yoga poses such as downward dog, warrior poses, and tree pose target the core, arms, legs, and back, while Pilates exercises like the hundred, leg circles, and the teaser focus on strengthening the core muscles. By incorporating these exercises into a regular workout routine, individuals can see significant improvements in their strength and muscle tone.

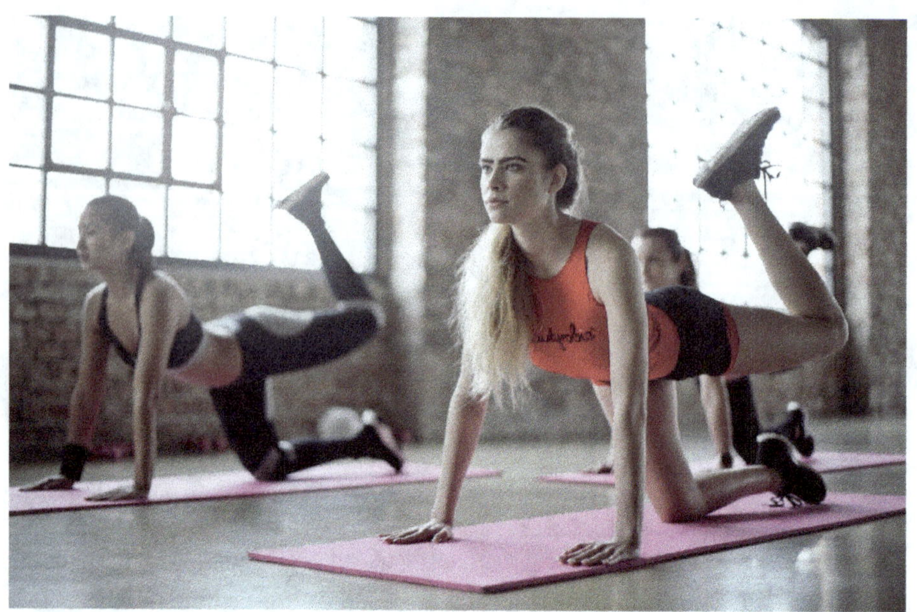

In addition to improving strength and flexibility, yoga and Pilates can also help individuals improve their posture and reduce the risk of injury. Many people who struggle with weight loss also struggle with poor posture, which can lead to back pain, neck pain, and other issues. By practicing yoga and Pilates regularly, individuals can strengthen their core muscles, improve their alignment, and reduce the strain on their joints, leading to better overall health and well-being.

Overall, incorporating yoga and Pilates into a weight loss and fitness routine can have a positive impact on both physical and mental health. These practices not only help individuals build strength, flexibility, and muscle tone, but they also provide a sense of calm and relaxation that can be beneficial for those dealing with stress, anxiety, or depression. By making yoga and Pilates a regular part of their lifestyle change journey, individuals can see lasting results and enjoy a healthier, happier life.

Chapter 9: Weightlifting and Muscle Building

How Weightlifting Aids in Weight Loss

Weightlifting is often overlooked as a tool for weight loss, but it can be incredibly effective in helping individuals shed unwanted pounds and keep them off for good. Many people think of cardio as the go-to exercise for weight loss, but strength training is just as important, if not more so, in achieving long-term success. In this subchapter, we will explore how weightlifting aids in weight loss and why it should be an essential part of any fitness routine for those looking to change their lifestyle and improve their health.

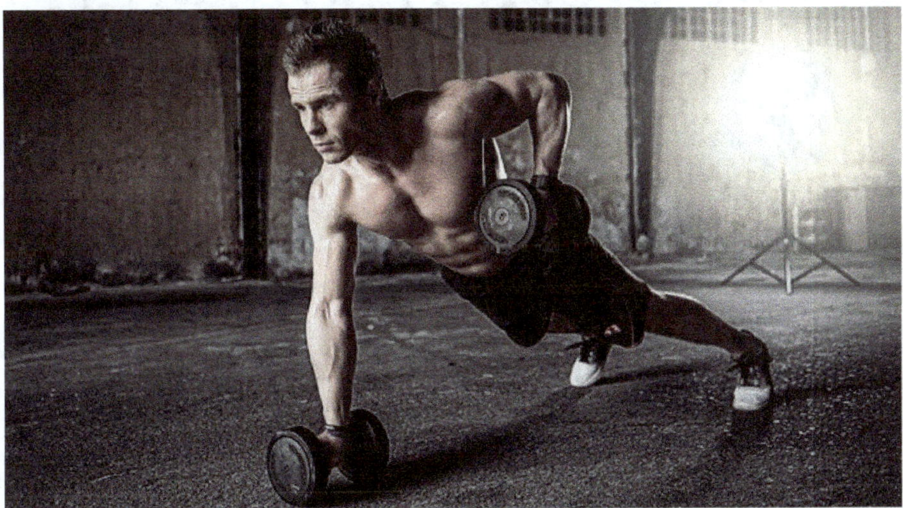

One of the key ways that weightlifting helps with weight loss is by increasing muscle mass. When you lift weights, you are not only burning calories during your workout, but you are also building lean muscle mass. Muscle burns more calories at rest than fat does, so the more muscle you have, the higher your resting metabolic rate will be. This means that you will burn more calories throughout the day, even when you are not actively exercising, making it easier to maintain a healthy weight.

In addition to boosting your metabolism, weightlifting can also help to sculpt your body and improve your overall physique. As you build muscle and burn fat, you will notice changes in your body composition, with a more toned and defined appearance. This can be incredibly motivating and rewarding, helping you to stay on track with your weight loss goals and maintain your progress over time.

Furthermore, weightlifting can improve your strength and endurance, making it easier to perform everyday tasks and activities. As you get stronger, you may find that you have more energy and stamina, allowing you to be more active and burn even more calories throughout the day. This can lead to further weight loss and improvements in your overall fitness level, setting you up for long-term success in maintaining a healthy lifestyle.

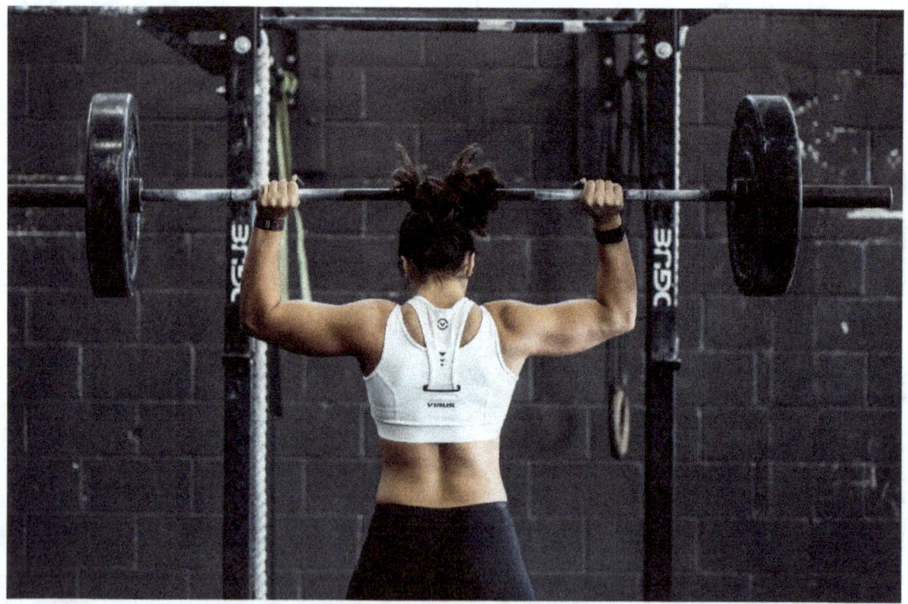

Overall, incorporating weightlifting into your fitness routine is essential for anyone looking to lose weight and keep it off. It offers a wide range of benefits, from boosting your metabolism and burning calories to sculpting your body and improving your strength and endurance. By including weightlifting in your workouts and focusing on building lean muscle mass, you can achieve lasting results and transform your body and health for the better. So don't underestimate the power of weightlifting in your weight loss journey – it may just be the missing piece to help you reach your goals and live a healthier, happier life.

Basic Weightlifting Exercises for Beginners

In this subchapter, we will cover some basic weightlifting exercises that are perfect for beginners looking to kickstart their fitness journey. Weightlifting is a great way to build strength, increase muscle mass, and boost metabolism, making it an essential component of any weight loss program.

First and foremost, it's important to start with light weights and focus on proper form to prevent injury. Begin with exercises such as squats, lunges, and deadlifts to target multiple muscle groups and improve overall strength. These compound movements are highly effective for burning calories and building lean muscle mass.

Another key exercise for beginners is the bench press, which targets the chest, shoulders, and triceps. Start with a light weight and gradually increase as you build strength. Remember to keep your core engaged and maintain proper form throughout the movement to maximize results.

For the back muscles, try exercises such as bent-over rows and lat pulldowns. These movements help improve posture, strengthen the upper back, and prevent injuries. Focus on squeezing the muscles and controlling the weight to get the most out of each rep.

To target the arms, include bicep curls and tricep extensions in your routine. These isolation exercises help tone and define the muscles, giving your arms a more sculpted appearance. Start with light weights and gradually increase as you gain strength and endurance.

In conclusion, incorporating basic weightlifting exercises into your fitness routine can help you achieve your weight loss goals and transform your body.

Remember to start slow, focus on proper form, and gradually increase the intensity as you progress. With dedication and consistency, you will see improvements in strength, muscle tone, and overall fitness level.

Incorporating Weightlifting into Your Workout Routine

Incorporating weightlifting into your workout routine can be a game-changer when it comes to losing weight and keeping it off. Many people think that weightlifting is just for bodybuilders or those looking to bulk up, but the truth is that it can be incredibly beneficial for anyone looking to improve their overall fitness and health. If you're feeling low motivated or stuck in a rut with your current workout routine, adding in some weightlifting exercises could be just what you need to see real results.

One of the great things about incorporating weightlifting into your workout routine is that it can help you build lean muscle mass, which can in turn boost your metabolism and help you burn more calories throughout the day. This can be especially helpful for those looking to lose weight and keep it off, as building muscle can help you achieve a toned and sculpted physique.

If you're new to weightlifting, don't be intimidated. There are plenty of beginner-friendly exercises that you can incorporate into your routine, such as squats, lunges, and bicep curls. These exercises can help you build strength and improve your overall fitness level, all while helping you achieve your weight loss goals.

In addition to helping you lose weight, weightlifting can also improve your overall health and well-being. Regular strength training can help reduce your risk of chronic diseases such as heart disease, diabetes, and osteoporosis. It can also improve your balance and coordination, which can help prevent falls as you age.

So if you're looking to shake up your workout routine and see real results, consider incorporating weightlifting into your regimen. Whether you're a mom, dad, or just someone looking to make a lifestyle change, adding in some weightlifting exercises could be the key to achieving your fitness and weight loss goals. With a combination of weightlifting, cardio, and proper nutrition, you can create a well-rounded workout routine that will help you lose weight and keep it off for good.

Chapter 10: Outdoor Workouts for Weight Loss

Advantages of Outdoor Workouts

Outdoor workouts offer numerous advantages for individuals looking to lose weight and maintain a healthy lifestyle. One of the main benefits of exercising outdoors is the fresh air and natural surroundings, which can help boost mood and motivation. Being surrounded by nature can also reduce stress levels and improve overall well-being, making outdoor workouts a great option for those feeling stuck in a rut or lacking motivation.

In addition to the mental health benefits, outdoor workouts can also provide a more challenging and varied workout compared to indoor exercises. The uneven terrain and elements such as wind and sun can add an extra level of difficulty to your workout, helping you burn more calories and build strength. Whether you're hiking up a steep trail, running on the beach, or doing bodyweight exercises in a park, outdoor workouts can help you push past your limits and achieve your fitness goals.

Another advantage of outdoor workouts is the flexibility and convenience they offer. With no need for expensive gym memberships or equipment, you can easily fit in a workout whenever and wherever it suits you. This can be especially helpful for busy Moms, Dads, or anyone struggling to find time for exercise in their daily routine. Outdoor workouts also provide a great opportunity to involve the whole family, making it a fun and interactive way to stay active together.

Outdoor workouts can also be a great way to mix up your routine and prevent boredom. Instead of being stuck in a crowded gym or following the same workout videos at home, you can explore new locations and try different types of exercises outdoors. Whether you're into high-intensity interval training, bodyweight exercises, strength training, cardio workouts, or yoga and Pilates, there are endless possibilities for outdoor workouts to keep you engaged and motivated.

Overall, outdoor workouts offer a holistic approach to fitness and weight loss, combining physical activity with the benefits of nature and fresh air. By incorporating outdoor workouts into your routine, you can not only achieve your weight loss goals but also improve your mental and emotional well-being. So, if you're looking for a fun, challenging, and convenient way to change your lifestyle and maintain a healthy weight, consider taking your workout outdoors and experience the many advantages it has to offer.

Sample Outdoor Workout Ideas for Weight Loss

Are you tired of the same old gym routine and looking for fun and effective ways to lose weight? Look no further than outdoor workouts! Exercising outdoors not only provides a change of scenery but also allows you to enjoy the fresh air and vitamin D from the sun. In this subchapter, we will explore some sample outdoor workout ideas specifically designed for weight loss to help you achieve your fitness goals and maintain a healthy lifestyle.

High-intensity interval training (HIIT) workouts are a great way to burn calories and boost your metabolism. HIIT involves short bursts of intense exercise followed by brief periods of rest or lower-intensity exercise. This type of workout is perfect for busy individuals who want to maximize their time and see results quickly. Outdoor HIIT workouts can include sprints, jumping jacks, burpees, and mountain climbers. These exercises can be done in a park, on a trail, or even in your backyard.

Bodyweight exercises are another fantastic option for weight loss. These exercises use your own body weight as resistance, making them convenient and accessible for all fitness levels. Squats, lunges, push-ups, and planks are just a few examples of bodyweight exercises that can help you build muscle and burn fat. Outdoor bodyweight workouts can be done at a local park or on a beach, allowing you to enjoy nature while getting in a great workout.

Strength training is essential for weight loss and overall health. Building muscle not only increases your metabolism but also improves your strength and endurance. If you are new to strength training, outdoor workouts can be a great way to get started. You can use resistance bands, dumbbells, or even rocks and logs as weights. Outdoor strength training workouts can include exercises like bicep curls, shoulder presses, and squats. Remember to focus on proper form and gradually increase the weight as you get stronger.

Cardio workouts are key for burning fat and improving cardiovascular health. Running, cycling, and jumping rope are excellent options for outdoor cardio workouts. These activities can be done in a park, on a trail, or around your neighborhood. Outdoor cardio workouts not only help you shed pounds but also boost your mood and energy levels. Mix up your routine by trying different activities and exploring new outdoor locations to keep things interesting and challenging.

In addition to regular exercise, proper nutrition is essential for weight loss and overall well-being. Make sure to fuel your body with healthy and balanced meals to support your fitness goals. Meal planning can help you stay on track and avoid unhealthy food choices. Consider consulting with a nutritionist or dietitian for personalized advice and guidance. Remember, consistency is key when it comes to lifestyle change and weight loss. Incorporating outdoor workouts into your routine can help you stay motivated, break through plateaus, and achieve lasting results. So lace up your sneakers, grab a water bottle, and start sweating it out in the great outdoors!

Staying Motivated with Outdoor Exercise

Staying motivated with outdoor exercise can be a game-changer for those looking to lose weight and keep it off. The fresh air, sunshine, and change of scenery can provide a much-needed boost to your workout routine. Whether you're a busy mom, dad, or simply someone who has been feeling stuck in a rut, incorporating outdoor exercise into your lifestyle can help you stay on track and motivated towards reaching your fitness goals.

One of the key benefits of outdoor exercise is the variety it offers. Instead of being confined to a gym setting, you have the freedom to explore different environments and try new activities. Whether it's going for a run in the park, biking on a scenic trail, or doing bodyweight exercises at the beach, the options are endless. This variety can help prevent boredom and keep you engaged in your workouts, making it easier to stay motivated and consistent.

Additionally, outdoor exercise can provide a mental break from the stresses of daily life. Being surrounded by nature can have a calming effect on the mind, helping to reduce anxiety and improve overall mental well-being. This can be especially beneficial for parents who are juggling multiple responsibilities and need a moment to focus on themselves and their health.

If you're feeling low on motivation, consider finding a workout buddy or joining a group fitness class outdoors. Exercising with others can provide accountability and support, making it more likely that you'll stick to your fitness routine. Not to mention, the social aspect can make your workouts more enjoyable and help you build a sense of community with like-minded individuals.

In conclusion, incorporating outdoor exercise into your lifestyle can be a powerful tool for staying motivated and reaching your weight loss goals. Whether you're trying high-intensity interval training (HIIT) workouts, bodyweight exercises, or simply going for a walk in nature, the key is to find activities that you enjoy and that fit your schedule. With dedication and consistency, you can transform your lifestyle and achieve lasting results. So, lace up your sneakers, step outside, and let the great outdoors be your fitness playground.

Congratulations on taking the first step towards a healthier, stronger, and more vibrant you! As you reach the end of this book, remember that your journey to fitness is just beginning. Every workout, every healthy meal, and every positive choice you make brings you closer to your goals.

It's natural to encounter obstacles along the way, but don't let them derail your progress. Embrace challenges as opportunities for growth and remember that setbacks are temporary. Stay focused on your vision, stay committed to your plan, and never underestimate the power of consistency.

Believe in yourself and your ability to succeed. You are capable of achieving amazing things when you put your mind to it. Trust the process, celebrate your victories, and keep pushing forward, one step at a time.

Above all, remember that fitness is not just about physical strength—it's about resilience, determination, and the relentless pursuit of your best self. You have the strength within you to overcome any obstacle and achieve your dreams.

So keep moving, keep striving, and keep believing in yourself. Your journey is unique, your potential is limitless, and your future is bright. Here's to a lifetime of health, happiness, and endless possibilities. You've got this!"